Palliative Care Resuscitation

MADELINE BASS
Palliative Care Nurse Specialist
RGN, MIFA, BSc (Hons)

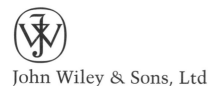

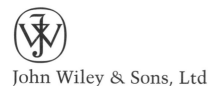

John Wiley & Sons, Ltd

Copyright © 2006   John Wiley & Sons Ltd
    The Atrium, Southern Gate, Chichester,
    West Sussex PO19 8SQ, England
    Telephone (+44) 1243 779777

Email (for orders and customer service enquiries): cs-books@wiley.co.uk

Visit our Home Page on www.wiley.com

Other Wiley Editorial Offices

John Wiley & Sons Inc., 111 River Street, Hoboken, NJ 07030, USA

Jossey-Bass, 989 Market Street, San Francisco, CA 94103-1741, USA

Wiley-VCH Verlag GmbH, Boschstr. 12, D-69469 Weinheim, Germany

John Wiley & Sons Australia Ltd, 42 McDougall Street, Milton, Queensland 4064, Australia

John Wiley & Sons (Asia) Pte Ltd, 2 Clementi Loop #02-01, Jin Xing Distripark, Singapore 129809

John Wiley & Sons Canada Ltd, 6045 Freemont Blvd, Mississauga, Ontario, L5R 4J3, Canada

Wiley also publishes its books in a variety of electronic formats. Some content that appears in print may not be available in electronic books.

Library of Congress Cataloging-in-Publication Data

Bass, Madeline.
    Palliative care resuscitation / Madeline Bass.
        p.   ;   cm.
    Includes bibliographical references and index.
    ISBN-13: 978-0-470-01977-1 (pbk. : alk. paper)
    ISBN-10: 0-470-01977-8 (pbk. : alk. paper)
    1. Palliative treatment.   2. Terminal care.   3. Resuscitation.   I. Title.
    [DNLM: 1. Cardiopulmonary Resuscitation.   2. Advance Directives.
3. Guideline Adherence.   4. Nurse's Role.   5. Palliative Care – methods.
6. Resuscitation Orders – ethics. WG 205 B317p 2006]
    R726.8.B37 2006
    616′.029 – dc22   2006008577

A catalogue record for this book is available from the British Library

ISBN-13 978-0-470-01977-1
ISBN-10 0-470-01977-8

Typeset in 10/12pt Times by SNP Best-set Typesetter Ltd., Hong Kong
Printed and bound in Great Britain by TJ International Ltd, Padstow, Cornwall

This book is printed on acid-free paper responsibly manufactured from sustainable forestry in which at least two trees are planted for each one used for paper production.

Contents

This book is dedicated to my husband, Andrew, without whose support I would not have achieved anything in life, and would not have finished this book. Thanks for all the shopping, cleaning and ironing you have done to enable me to have time to do this.

Preface

I feel very privileged to have been given the chance to write this book, something I have always wanted to do but never thought I would.

The subject of resuscitation in palliative care has been one close to my heart for a few years now, since carrying out some research for my dissertation. The research was based on oncology nurses' perceptions of resuscitation status for oncology patients. Although only a small study it generated some interesting points and clarified certain issues. From this I became involved in our Trust's patient information group for producing patient and family carer's information on resuscitation. From this, I have been able to undertake teaching sessions on the subject, not only within my own Trust but also to others.

The study and learning that writing this book has generated for me has given me even greater knowledge and insight into the subject of resuscitation in palliative care and I hope this book, written mainly for nurses and other allied health professionals, will fire up others to take this forward within their own Trusts and areas of patient care. The subject is by no means a cut and dried one; indeed, there are many grey areas. But I hope this book will aim to resolve some of the questions and ethical considerations the topic generates and encourage all healthcare workers that it is an area of major importance.

Certain phrases have been used throughout the book which may not be familiar to the reader. For instance, the phrase 'Do Not Attempt Resuscitation' (DNAR) has been used for people who are given an order not to receive cardiopulmonary resuscitation. This is the phrase recommended to be used by the resuscitation guidelines, for those patients who should not receive it. The term 'family carers' has been used for anyone who is a friend, relative or next of kin to the patient. This is now the correct term for any significant other who is involved in caring for the patient. And, yes, I have used the term patient, and not client, within the book, for this reason: I do not feel any person who develops a palliative illness is a client, since the word *client* generates visions, to me, of someone who has entered into a contract with someone else through choice. I am sure most, if not all, palliative care patients would not choose to be in the health status they are, hence the use of the word *patient*.

I have chosen some case studies to attempt to highlight certain issues discussed in the chapters. These case studies are entirely fictitious and have only been used as a teaching resource.

Finally, I hope you will enjoy the book as much as I have enjoyed the learning experience and the writing of it. I hope it will enable you to see the value of life and of a good death, and how important palliative care and its principles are. I wish you all a long and happy career in patient care.

Madeline Bass
2006

Acknowledgements

Where to start, I don't know! So many people have been involved in supporting me through this writing process, so for anyone I leave out please forgive me and please realise I am very grateful to you. First, to my long-suffering work colleagues, who have encouraged and supported me, made me many cups of tea when I have been discouraged about the book, and have told me lots of jokes to keep me going. Thanks for being such a great bunch, Nicky, Phil, Hilary, Sally and Libby. I hope we will work together for many years to come. Thanks also to Alison and Lisa, my managers, who have taken an interest in this as well. Thanks to the hospital library staff for all their help over the past year. Thanks to my parents and parents-in-law, who have always asked me how things are progressing and have listened to my whining and complaints when things have not been too easy. Thanks to my friends, Lisa, Liz and Martin, Sarah and Phil, Dave and Kirstie, Helen and Stuart, Kerry and Sue, who have been so fantastic and treated me like a major author. I know they are champing at the bit to read the end result! Thanks to my dog, Mac, for making me take him out for walks when I have been fed up, and for always being a loyal companion. The biggest thanks go to my husband, Andrew, who has been a full-time house-husband as well as full-time worker, and has given me plenty of hugs and cups of tea to help me through. Thank you for all your love, care and humour, which has got me through. I am so proud to be your wife, friend and soulmate.

1 The history of cardiopulmonary resuscitation

The development of modern cardiopulmonary resuscitation (CPR) has influenced today's Western society into feeling that there is control over death at any time. Western society and Western medicine zealously pursues immortality, and because medical research has discovered cures for diseases which decades ago would have killed many, patients have literally been brought back from the brink of death with the new medical technological advances that have been made, such as genetically engineered drugs, organ transplantation and life-support machines and devices. Yet death remains an everyday occurrence.

This feeling of control over death has been reinforced by the media, which has portrayed CPR as dignified, easy to do, appropriate for all and usually successful (BMA *et al.*, 2001). The media, including Hollywood, also portrays death itself as violent, sudden or romantic (Cooley, 2000). The many medical and nursing dramas on television often include incidences of CPR and its portrayal is mostly far removed from reality. Western society is fascinated by death, disease and illness, something which the media has profited from, and this fascination includes CPR. Unfortunately, with CPR, as with many other medical procedures, there is a stark difference between what is portrayed by the media and reality. This leaves the public with little true understanding of what CPR really involves, and often leaves people puzzled, bewildered and angry when it is not appropriate for themselves or their relative.

However, modern CPR (i.e. closed chest cardiac massage, defibrillation and mouth-to-mouth resuscitation) has only been used since 1960. It is amazing how something so relatively new is widely accepted in hospitals and the community alike, is seen as normal and as something to be expected. CPR is the one procedure in medicine for which consent is sought against it, not for it. The need for CPR is the only situation which imposes an apparent duty on health professionals to discuss a futile treatment without request from the patient, and equally, a situation where health professionals appear relieved of the obligation to discuss a treatment they plan to implement, as with non-futile CPR (Thorns, 2000).

Cardiopulmonary arrest can be defined as when a person's heart and breathing stop, or, 'Loss of consciousness with absence of circulation, accompanied by absent or gasping respirations' (Quinn, 1998). When this happens it is some-times possible to reverse respiratory and cardiac arrest, using CPR which might include:

- repeatedly pushing down firmly on the chest
- using electric shocks to try and restart the heart
- 'mouth to mouth' breathing
- inflating the lungs through a mask over the nose and mouth or tube inserted into the windpipe. (BMA *et al.*, 2001)

The aims of CPR are to restart the heart and breathing to the extent that the body can support itself.

The British Medical Association (BMA), the Royal College of Nursing (RCN) and the Resuscitation Council UK (RCUK) have produced some very comprehensive guidelines concerning cardiac and respiratory resuscitation (BMA *et al.*, 2001). These guidelines state that resuscitation can be attempted on any person whose cardiac or respiratory functions cease; however, it must be accepted that failure of these functions is part of the dying process and for everyone there comes a time when death is inevitable. It is important there-fore to identify those patients for whom cardiopulmonary arrest is caused by a terminal event, and for whom CPR would not be appropriate, in order to ensure that they have a dignified death.

The development of CPR itself has had some rather bizarre steps along the way. Resuscitation of the dead is a recurrent theme in ancient mythology, and artificial respiration by midwives helping newborn babies to breathe is docu-mented in the Book of Kings (in the Bible). In the early ages the heat method was used to try and revive people, hoping to warm the cooling body and restore heartbeat and breathing; this involved placing hot coals on the victim's thorax. It proved successful in some cases of hypothermia and unconscious-ness but not in victims of actual cardiopulmonary arrest. In the 1500s the bellows method became popular; this involved the use of fire bellows which were placed in the victim's mouth and used to inflate the lungs. The occasional success of this method led to the design of the bag–valve–mask resuscitators used today. However, the authorities at the time were not yet aware of the need to hyper-extend the airway in order to allow good air entry into the lungs, so the method was not as successful as it may have been. The early 1700s saw the use of the fumigation method, one which was at times successful but it is difficult to say why. It was initially used by the North American Indians and then by the American colonists and later introduced to England in 1767. The method involved filling the removed bladder of an animal with tobacco smoke and then blowing this smoke into the victim's rectum. In 1744 Tossach used mouth-to-mouth artificial respiration on a drowned person, but this method was abandoned in favour of more mechanical methods. In 1770 the inversion method became popular. This was when the victim's ankles were tied together with a rope, which was then fixed to a pulley. The victim was hoisted up by the ankles and alternately raised and lowered in an attempt to get air in and out of the chest cavity.

In the late 1700s, societies for preventing sudden death began to appear throughout Europe, for example the Dutch Society for Recovery of Drowned Persons, founded in 1767, and the Royal Human Society in Great Britain, founded in 1774. These societies practised some of the resuscitation techniques of the time, such as laying the body over a wine barrel and rolling the thorax backwards and forwards to cause chest compressions (late 1700s) or placing the person on the back of a trotting horse so that the motions also reproduced chest compressions (early 1800s). This latter method was initially used by American lifeguards on the beaches but was stopped by the 'Citizens for Clean Beaches Campaigners', about 1815. In the early 1800s the Russians adopted the ice method, encasing the victim's body in ice and snow in the hope of slowing the body's metabolism. Unfortunately, the method omitted to cool the head, which is also needed in order to slow the body's metabolism.

The publication of Mary Shelley's book, *Frankenstein, or the Modern Prometheus*, in 1818 caused artificial respiration and CPR to disappear for many years. The story of a mad scientist bringing life to a dead body did nothing to enhance the image of CPR.

In 1898 Tuffier and Halllon performed open chest cardiac massage successfully and this then became the popular method of cardiac resuscitation until the 1950s. In 1899 Provost and Batelli used alternate-current open-chest cardiac defibrillation on dogs with induced ventricular fibrillation with success. In the early 1900s Crile described closed-chest cardiac massage and recognised the importance of achieving adequate coronary perfusion pressure, and also the value of adrenaline.

The increasing use of electricity in the early twentieth century allowed the development of defibrillation for ventricular fibrillation. High fatality rates among electrical workers lead Edison to support the development of an electrical defibrillator by Hooker, Kouwenhoven and Langworthy. Wiggers also made significant contributions to the understanding of the pathophysiology of ventricular fibrillation at this time. Beck reported the first successful case of open defibrillation in 1947, and Zoll reported successful closed-chest defibrillation using alternate current in 1956.

In the late 1950s doctors Safar and Elam demonstrated that mouth-to-mouth rescue breathing was superior to the mechanical techniques previously used. The interest in closed-chest cardiac massage was rekindled around this time as well. Bahnson successfully used this technique to resuscitate a small child in 1958, and in the 1950s the US military began an aggressive public campaign on the use of mouth-to-mouth resuscitation, which they had used successfully in World War Two. American lifeguards were instructed on how to perform mouth-to-mouth resuscitation whilst in the water, using flotation aids.

Further research was carried out on cardiac defibrillation in the 1960s. Dr Frank Partridge was responsible for the first portable defibrillators being put into ambulances in 1963: at that time they were size of a small refrigerator, and difficult to use (hard to believe as today defibrillators are easily portable, and increasingly available for use by the public).

CPR as we know it today was fully developed by Kouwenhoven *et al.* in 1960, and combined mouth-to-mouth resuscitation, defibrillation and closed-chest cardiac massage. This research was fully reported in the *Journal of the American Medical Association* (JAMA) in 1960. The article outlined the crucial aspect of this whole technique (using either open- or closed-chest cardiac massage), which was that the patient received oxygenated blood that would then be transported to the brain by minimal blood circulation, reducing anoxia and its effects on the brain and body. It described the team's previous research on closed-chest compressions in cats and dogs and the noted positive blood pressure changes this technique induced. This method was then applied to humans, the anatomy of the thorax lending itself to such chest compressions: the sternum, vertebrae and ribs provide an enclosed area with support, allowing the heart to be compressed when pressure is applied correctly, and then to relax when this pressure is removed, thus allowing the heart to fill with blood again. This method was also meant to allow some lung ventilation and the article advocated concentrating mainly on the chest compressions if a person was attempting CPR on a patient by themself. This method of CPR was trialled at the John Hopkins Hospital, in the USA, over a nine-month period. Twenty patients, aged between two months and 80 years, were all resuscitated successfully, and 14 of them lived to the time the article was written 10 months later. Five cases were reported in detail, four of which needed resuscitation during surgery and one of which was admitted to the emergency room in ventricular fibrillation. There are no details given of which of the 20 patients survived, or anything to suggest why.

On the surface, CPR sounded fantastic: the answer to every doctor's need, helping them to overcome death and disease more than ever. Unfortunately, all the cases reported were sudden, traumatic events, nothing to do with palliative care or death from terminal illness. The application of this method of CPR so readily to nearly all areas of medicine is frighteningly intense, and has probably been influenced heavily by medical paternalism (i.e. medical staff take the dominant role in care and treatment decisions). Ironically, at a similar time, Dame Cicely Saunders was one becoming of the first pioneers of palliative care, and the hospice movement.

In the 1970s CPR was introduced to the public, and in the past few years it has been added as mandatory to all first aid training as well as to all medical and nurse training, with mandatory yearly updates required of all clinical staff. It is available world wide and resuscitation teams are found in every general hospital. It is a widely accepted and expected management of cardiac arrest, and is regulated and advised by the Resuscitation Council in the UK, Europe and worldwide. These councils work in conjunction with medical and nursing councils worldwide in order to update CPR guidelines and training as required.

The history and development of CPR provides some insight into its ongoing importance in medicine; however, this must be balanced with appropriate use, likely success and possible side effects.

2 CPR versus active treatment in palliative care

Cardiopulmonary resuscitation (CPR) includes mouth-to-mouth resuscitation, closed-chest cardiac massage and defibrillation. The aim of CPR is to support the body's circulation to prevent the effects of anoxia until the circulation can be restored, or until such efforts are seen to be futile. However, there are other medical treatments and interventions which can be used to support these body systems if they begin to weaken, but which will not support cardiac and respiratory function if it has ceased altogether (BMA *et al.*, 2001). These are collectively known as 'active treatment', and they include many things to try and prevent the function of the heart and lungs from ceasing, such as antibiotics, intravenous fluids, diuretics, blood transfusions and so on. Active treatment may be appropriate in situations where CPR is not, or when it has been refused. When discussing CPR with patients and their family carers it is important that the distinction is made between CPR and active treatment. Explanations should be given that 'Do Not Attempt Resuscitation' (DNAR), sometimes called 'Not for Resuscitation' (NFR), does not mean 'no treatment'.

Even if active treatment is not appropriate for certain patients, palliative care and good, supportive, holistic nursing care can often reassure patients and their family carers, and reinforce the importance of a dignified 'good' death. To prevent confusion the resuscitation guidelines suggest that one phrase is used when patients are 'not for resuscitation': 'Do Not Attempt Resuscitation' (DNAR) and that other phrases are used when considering active or alternative treatment. The guidelines are corroborated by the American Medical Association.

Willard (2002) argues that there is a lack of clarity about what palliative care is, and this is coupled with our increased ability to extend life. This situation seems to be creating substantial and unacknowledged difficulties for some healthcare professionals. For example, Willard says that healthcare professionals could question the extent to which they are able to reconcile two sometimes conflicting aims: the desire to extend survival by providing what can be quite aggressive treatment and the desire to promote a good quality of life. Does this dilemma, therefore, have implications for the way professionals make decisions and care for patients? Willard feels it does – by professionals tending to oversimplify the patient's situation.

The term 'Do Not Resuscitate' can have great emotional overtones. Thus the BMA in the resuscitation guidelines (BMA *et al.*, 2001) has advised that the phrase should be 'Do Not *Attempt* Resuscitation', since this seems less medically paternalistic and implies that other interventions may be tried instead where appropriate. What resuscitation should be aiming for is the revival of someone for whom cardiac or respiratory arrest was unex-pected, and for whom CPR would be appropriate. Resuscitation is simply what it says, it is not resurrection (Saunders, 2001). Life does end for all living things, and all medical and healthcare professionals need to be brave enough, and sensible enough, to identify those who have reached the end of life, and those for whom life could be appropriately lengthened for the correct reasons.

Palliative care is an approach that improves quality of life for patients who have life-threatening, incurable, progressive disease, and their family carers, through the prevention and relief of suffering, by the use of early identification and impeccable assessment and treatment of pain and other problems, including psychosocial and spiritual issues (WHO, 2002). The word *palliative* comes from the Latin *palliare* meaning 'to cloak', or 'shield'. The term 'supportive care' is sometimes used for the universal, general palliative care that every healthcare professional should be capable of providing, regardless of diagnosis, discipline or speciality they are working in. It is also the right of every cancer and palliative patient to receive this, and the duty of every professional to provide it (Regnard and Kindlen, 2002).

The terms 'palliative care', 'hospice care' and 'terminal care' are often used interchangeably (Doyle, 1994). Palliative care is not exclusively terminal care: terminal care is only one phase of palliative care and usually refers to the final stage of a person's life, normally the last few weeks or days. It is, however, generally recognised that palliative care is for people whose disease is not responsive to curative treatment (WHO, 2002). The terminal phase of an illness can be difficult to recognise, therefore care of the dying starts from the time the incurable diagnosis has been made (Lugton, 2002). Palliative care is a relatively new science and has become a speciality since the late 1980s. It now includes support for patients with non-malignant diagnoses, thus extending and applying the skills and symptom control knowledge of the specialist palliative care practitioner to providing support and symptom control advice and knowledge for other incurable diseases which may have equally distressing symptoms and poor prognoses.

It may be difficult to recognise when a disease becomes palliative, and this mostly occurs when previous treatment methods no longer have as much effect, or result in more side-effects than benefits. The care of dying people takes place mainly in hospitals, as most deaths occur there (57%; Office of National Statistics, 2003), in hospices, where a small number of deaths occur

(Field and James, 1993), and in community settings such as residential and nursing homes, community hospitals or at home.

Palliative care is governed by certain principles which guide the care given. It:

- provides relief from pain and other distressing symptoms
- affirms life and regards death as a normal process
- intends neither to hasten or postpone death
- integrates the psychological and spiritual aspects of patient care
- offers a support system to help the family cope during the patient's illness and in bereavement
- uses a team approach to address the needs of patients and their families, including counselling if indicated
- will enhance quality of life and may positively influence the course of the illness
- is applicable early in the course of the illness, in conjunction with other therapies that may prolong life, such as chemotherapy or radiation therapy, and includes investigations needed to better understand and manage distressing clinical complications (WHO, 2004).

Other principles of palliative care promote:

- quality of life: palliative care tries to enhance this as much as is realistically possible
- patient choices: patient autonomy is respected and encouraged as much as possible
- open communication
- looking after the whole person (holistic care), which includes physical, emotional, psychological, spiritual and intellectual issues
- looking after the whole family because the patient is not an isolated unit but part of a whole social unit; patients' disease, and its effects may have catastrophic influences on this social unit and its dynamics
- involving support from the whole multi-disciplinary team: this includes professionals in the hospital and community, such as doctors, nurses, palliative care specialists, hospice services, dieticians, physiotherapists, occupational therapists and chaplaincy (Regnard and Kindlen, 2002).

It can be seen from the definition of palliative care and its principles that CPR is not always in the patient's best interests, especially not in the terminal phases of an illness. CPR was initially designed by Kouwenhoven *et al.* (1960) for sudden, unpredictable cardiac events or traumatic situations in which cardiac arrest has occurred as a sudden, initial event. Everyone who dies technically experiences a cardiac arrest because their heart stops. In terminal illness, cardiac arrest occurs as the last event in an illness or disease. The body has slowly shut down and no longer requires the same nutritional support, produces less urine and faeces, and the heart and lungs become much weaker and less able to cope with the body's circulatory fluid and lung mucous. This can often result in a build up of terminal secretions ('death rattle'). Often, patients approaching death can show signs of deterioration over a period of hours, days or weeks. Such signs can include needing to rest and sleep more often, increasing lethargy, decreasing or non-existent appetite, weight loss, changes in respiratory status, skin colour, low body temperature and low blood pressure. Because of this it seems unfair to use resuscitation techniques on those in this situation: their whole body is failing, not just the heart and lungs. Resuscitation will not work for them. In such situations resuscitation will be futile. Instead, the aim should be for a 'good death': in other words, a holistic death which is dignified and where the patient is comfortable and well-supported physically by good nursing care; their symptoms are controlled and their emotional, spiritual, psychological and intellectual needs, and those of their family carers, are met.

Case study 1

Mrs Smith is an 80-year-old lady who has been admitted to hospital with right upper quadrant pain. She has had this pain for some months on and off, but thought it was probably gallstones. She felt her GP was making a huge fuss about this pain, although she did agree with him that she did look a funny colour, slightly jaundiced. She has also been losing weight for some time. Throughout the next few days in hospital Mrs Smith undergoes many different investigations but the results seem to take forever to come through. Her son lives away but has come to visit her one weekend, and is shocked by how much his mother has deteriorated in the few weeks since he has visited her last. He asks a doctor to speak to them both together one afternoon and try to explain at least what they think may be wrong with her. The doctor spends a long time with them both, and very carefully explains that Mrs Smith had been found to have liver secondaries, that is, spread of cancer, probably from a breast cancer primary tumour, and she has probably had this for some time. Mrs Smith confirms that her right breast has seemed unusual to look at, with puckered skin and a discharge from the nipple, for some time. The doctor states very clearly that this cancer is not curable because of the fact it has now spread to her liver. Because Mrs Smith has become very frail recently the doctor feels that the best treatment is to refer her to an oncologist, but explains quite clearly that she may only be offered some radiotherapy, and is not even sure that this would be appropriate. Mrs Smith asks how long he thinks she has, and the doctor explains he cannot give an accurate prognosis but that the family should prepare themselves, that time will be quite short, perhaps weeks, months at the outside. Mrs Smith and her son decide that she should go home to sort out a few things, and then return with her son to his own home to stay with him. The doctor says he will do what he can to ensure that the oncologist sees Mrs Smith as soon as possible in order that she can then return to her son's home. The oncologist is able to see Mrs Smith the next morning before her clinic, on the ward. She confirms that she feels Mrs Smith is too frail, and after further discussions about the side effects of chemotherapy and radiotherapy, and the possible success rates of these, Mrs Smith decides with her son she would rather be referred to her son's local oncology centre and to his local Macmillan nurses. The oncologist also speaks about resuscitation with her, openly and honestly. Mrs Smith feels that as she is really very unwell when she dies she does not want 'any heroics' performed; she wants to die peacefully with her family around her if possible. The oncologist takes the details of the son's local hospital and says she will telephone the oncology center there and fax the details about Mrs Smith's illness the next day. Mrs Smith then returns to her home with her son, where they stay for a few days, expedite an update on her will and sort through her valuables. Mrs Smith also tells her son what belongings she wants given to whom. Those few days are very emotional but both Mrs Smith and her son are able to share good memories and discuss their hopes and fears for her short future. Mrs Smith then returns to her son's home where, from the advice given by the oncologist, they contact his GP surgery, registering his mother with the practice and ask the community Macmillan nurses to make contact with them. The district nurse also makes contact with the family and leaves her number, explaining what her team may be able to assist with. The Macmillan nurse contacts them three days later and comes to assess Mrs Smith at her son's home. The nurse carries out a full assessment, including physical, emotional, social, psychological and spiritual enquiries of Mrs Smith and her son. During the conversation the nurse mentions the local hospice. Mrs Smith decides to visit during the following week, with her son. She is very impressed with the hospice and asks if she can stay at home with her son until she becomes too weak for him to care for her. She and her son enjoy another six weeks at home, and although Mrs Smith becomes much more frail during this time she and her son share some very special memories. The Macmillan nurse visits regularly and addresses Mrs Smith's symptoms of pain and nausea with the support of the local symptom control 'Hospice at Home' team. The district nurse also visits to monitor Mrs Smith in general and to give extra support, such as arranging carers to help when she begins to need help with personal hygiene. At the end of this time, the Macmillan nurse visits and agrees with Mrs Smith that it is time she is admitted to the hospice. On admission, two days later, one of the hospice doctors explains that as Mrs Smith is so frail, it will not be appropriate to attempt resuscitation when she dies as it would not be successful, but that other interventions such as good nursing care, good symptom relief and supportive nursing care will be given instead. Mrs Smith dies very peacefully in the company of her son six days later.

This case study highlights some of the main issues concerning palliative care patients. Although this case study appears quite idealistic, many palliative care patients' cases *do* happen like this. Notice how, in the first instance, when being given her diagnosis Mrs Smith had someone with her whom she could trust, her son, and who could support her. During this conversation the doctor was very honest with them both, and used words such as *cancer* and *not curable*, and also shied away from giving a prognosis as this can be so difficult to do accurately. The oncologist visited was very soon after the doctor had given Mrs Smith and her son her diagnosis. She was very honest with Mrs Smith and her son, and offered her only the interventions that she felt Mrs Smith would be able to tolerate but was very open about the side effects Mrs Smith would probably experience and what possible length this may add to her life. Because of this Mrs Smith was able to decide what she wanted to do in the future. She was followed up by her son's community services because he had been given the correct information needed to register his mother with his own GP surgery and he was also able to hand over some information to the GP about his mother's diagnosis. Mrs Smith's symptoms were dealt with as required by the community team and discussions about the hospice were appropriate: these were helpful to Mrs Smith's son, who may have found it hard to look after his mother alone. The discussions about resuscitation were carried out in front of Mrs Smith's son so that he understood the aims of her treatment and the aims of his mother's care, particularly at the hospice. He was allowed to stay during the last few days of her life so that he was with his mother when she died, which was what she had wanted.

It may seem that this case study is incredibly idealistic. However, nothing happened which could not, or should not, have happened. Yes, it seemed fortunate that there was a bed so soon at the hospice for her, but this can happen: most hospices will prioritise their beds to community patients before hospital patients, and because Mrs Smith was known to the local 'Hospice at Home' team they were able to access accurate, up-to-date information about her and believed she was in the last few days of life, it was therefore appropriate to admit her to the unit. What the reader needs to take away from this case study is that at no time was Mrs Smith made to feel unimportant, a waste of time or a waste of effort because of her age. The truth was told appropriately and this ensured that Mrs Smith and her son were fully aware of the aims of her treatment and care at all stages. Mrs Smith and her son were able to talk openly together about the future and to make all the arrangements they needed to before her death. Many similar instances in palliative care patients do occur; however, many do not. There are instances when patients and their family carers are not spoken to together, are not seen by a specialist quickly and do not have resuscitation discussed with them. Many patients do not have community teams support because accurate information is often not passed on quickly enough. Many do not get a bed at the local hospice in time, either because the referral is made too late in their illness, or because the patient and family do not understand the philosophy of hospice care and are too frightened to agree to admission. Mrs Smith's case could easily have gone differently.

Case study 2

Mrs Smith is an 80-year-old lady who has been admitted to hospital with right upper quadrant pain. Her son visits her and asks if he can speak to a doctor about his mother's illness and investigations. The doctor cannot get there straight away and visits late in the afternoon when Mrs Smith's son is tired and really just wants to go home. He tells Mrs Smith and her son that they have found some 'suspicious' lumps in her liver, probably due to a 'tumour' but that a 'specialist' would come to visit her to explain it further. The specialist (oncologist) visits a few days later (thus wasting time for Mrs Smith and her son). She assumes they have been told the diagnosis as the doctor recorded in the medical notes that he had spoken to her and her son together. She therefore speaks very openly to Mrs Smith and her son together about her cancer. Mrs Smith and her son are understandably quite shocked when the word 'cancer' is used and are both consequently very angry that the other doctor had not told them properly about her diagnosis. Because of the shock, Mrs Smith is not keen to discuss anything else at length, and simply wants to go to her home and then to her son's. The oncologist says she will refer Mrs Smith to her son's local oncology unit, which will send her an out patient appointment to discuss future care, but warns her that she may be too frail to have any treatment in the future. Resuscitation and prognosis are not discussed. Mrs Smith goes home, then to her son's. She is registered with her son's GP surgery and is visited by a district nurse. When this visit occurs Mrs Smith and her son are still very angry and are surprised that community Macmillan nurses and hospice are discussed. They do not feel this is appropriate as they are still waiting to see the local oncologist about possible treatments (they have not taken on board what the initial oncologist said about her probably being too frail to have any treatment in the future). In the next few days Mrs Smith becomes more unwell with increasing pain and shortness of breath, plus a chesty cough and temperature. She and her son are worried about this and request a visit from her GP, who offers admission to the hospice. They are still not happy to consider this as she has not been seen by the local oncologist. Despite her GP saying she is very ill and will be too unwell for any treatment Mrs Smith and her son request that she goes to hospital instead. Once admitted Mrs Smith is treated for a severe chest infection. The doctors speak to her son and explain she is very unwell and may not survive. They ask him if he would want his mother resuscitated if her heart or lungs stop working:

he agrees he would, as his mother still has not been seen by the local oncologist. His mother suffers a cardiac arrest in the night, which is actually a terminal event, but they attempt resuscitation because of her son's request: this fails and Mrs Smith dies shortly after admission without her son being with her.

This seems the complete antithesis of the first case study. Everything seems to go wrong, the patient and family do not understand what is going on, and Mrs Smith's son is then asked whether he would want his mother to be resuscitated. As hard as this might seem to some, and as normal as this may seem to others, this is not a satisfactory case study. Although there may not be many situations like this it is possible for many patients that poor information-giving occurs, as in the case of the doctor giving the initial bad news actually influencing every thing that happens after this. Note how his lack of truthfulness with Mrs Smith and her son mean that when the oncologist visits later on, the shock was too much for Mrs Smith and her son to be able to discuss future care and treatments properly because they needed time to digest the diagnosis. This case study should be used as an example of what can happen when inaccurate information and euphemisms are given to patients instead of using the correct terminology such as 'cancer' and 'incurable'. This lady died from metastatic cancer and an end-stage chest infection, after a failed attempt at resuscitation, which is still quite common in terminal care. Notice it was the son's request that this be carried out, and that he had been asked what he wanted: no advice was given as to how successful it would be to attempt resuscitation, or what the alternatives may be. As hard as it is to be honest with patients it is very important.

ARTIFICIAL HYDRATION, NUTRITION AND ACTIVE TREATMENT IN PALLIATIVE CARE

The subject of whether to use artificial hydration and nutrition in terminally ill patients, which could be included under the cloak of 'active treatment', has brought about different points of view. Rousseau (2000) states that many doctors and nurses feel food and fluid is always a basic need for human existence. However, although this is true, feeding terminally ill patients (either via nasogatric tube, nasojejunostomy, gastrostomy or parenteral routes, such as total parenteral nutrition [TPN]) has not been found to enhance or prolong life. Remember, tube feeding in no way resembles normal eating since it is a passive process that totally bypasses the sensation gained from oral feeding: there is no smell, taste or texture of feeling food in the mouth. Tube feeding can also have serious complications such as aspiration, nasal cartilage erosion and tube displacement, which may require an uncomfortable, perhaps even painful, replacement. It is important for healthcare professionals, patients and their family carers, to realise that weight loss and anorexia are part of the dying process and that the absence of tube feeding does not lead to death caused by starvation or dehydration; tube feeding does not lengthen life. In fact, it may encourage tumour growth (Rousseau, 2000).

It may be felt by some that artificial hydration is not required for various reasons, a feeling echoed by the National Council for Palliative Care (NCPC, 2002a). Reasons for this include that towards death a person's need for nutrition and fluid is lessened, and evidence suggests that artificial hydration in terminal illness neither prolongs life nor helps symptom control (Oliver, 1984; Billings, 1985; Rosner, 1987; Regnard and Mannix 1991; Printz, 1992; Andrews *et al.*, 1993; Burge, 1993; Sommerville, 1993; Tattersall, 1993; Twycross and Lichter, 1993; Craig, 1994; Fainsinger *et al.*, 1994; Dunphy *et al.*, 1995; Ellershaw *et al.*, 1995). Artificial hydration is not usually needed if good mouth care is given – think how quickly thirst is quenched when a few mouthfuls of drink are taken: it is some time before the fluid is actually absorbed by the body's system, yet almost immediately there is some relief from the thirst. Hence, it is felt that good mouth care can achieve the same results. The NCPC (2002a) continues that certain medications the terminally ill patient may be receiving such as morphine, can cause a dry mouth. Simply adding artificial hydration will not lessen this. The NCPC states that the use of artificial hydration to correct the correctable is appropriate, for example in hypercalcaemia, diarrhoea and delirium caused by electrolyte imbalance. Rousseau (2000) also argues that artificial hydration may cause a complication known as 'third spacing', which can cause peripheral and pulmonary oedema from low oncotic pressures, secondary to low blood albumen levels and poor nutritional status. It can also increase gastro-intestinal and pulmonary secretions, increase urinary output and in the end probably cause more patient discomfort then less (Printz, 1992; Kinzbrunner, 1995). If it is necessary to stop fluids for these reasons, it is helpful if the family carers are supported during this decision. If the family carers would prefer artificial fluids or nutrition to continue, sensitive explanation as to why they need to be stopped needs to be given. However, if there are no noticeable side effects from the fluids or nutrition already being given there is no reason to stop them. A blanket policy on artificial hydration is not an individual approach to patient care. Each terminally ill patient should be assessed according to their personal needs, present symptoms and family carers' concerns. Although caring for patients and their symptoms is important, each patient needs to be cared for as part of a social unit, and it must be recognised how doing this will affect those close to them. The patient is not a solitary item: he or she is part of a family unit which needs care as a whole.

Other thoughts concerning artificial hydration are that it is necessary, particularly when sedation is being used (Craig, 2002). This will help to flush out the toxins from the medications being used and prevents over-sedation. If the aim of sedation is to cause the patient to become unconscious, hydration must be used to prevent death through dehydration (unless, of course, there are contraindications for the use of fluids). Hydration may also be useful in patients experiencing delirium caused by abnormal electrolyte levels as it can increase the elimination of opioid metabolites. In the case of Mrs Smith above if she had been experiencing terminal agitation and required sedation, it would have been appropriate to give intravenous fluids unless she developed terminal secretions, at which point her body would not have been able to cope with the extra fluids. If the fluids had not been started, the nurses and doctors would need to observe Mrs Smith and try to prevent too much sedation being given: enough to hold the symptoms at bay but not enough to sedate her unnecessarily. This would be done by starting with a low dose of sedative in a syringe driver and giving extra doses as required, thus increasing the doses in the syringe driver according to requirements. If there were concerns about Mrs Smith needing hydration, particularly from the son's point of view, as long as there were no terminal secretions present some fluids could be commenced subcutaneously for Mrs Smith. However, good mouth care would also help prevent Mrs Smith experiencing thirst. Remember, the assessment of the need for fluids is an individual one, based on many issues.

Case study 3

Mrs Smith, the 80-year-old lady with metastatic breast cancer, when admitted to the hospice, looked physically dehydrated: her skin was very slack on the back of her hands and appeared dry on her face and arms. She also reported feeling very thirsty but was too frightened to drink very much as she was struggling to get to the toilet in time and did not want to give her son too much extra washing. She was quite muddled at times and felt nauseated. She also appeared very constipated: her son said she had been complaining of constipation for 'several days'. Some subcutaneous fluids were started by the hospice doctor and he stated that these were to prevent Mrs Smith feeling too thirsty. Her bloods were taken and showed she had a raised calcium level, which explained her nausea, constipation and confusion. These symptoms were treated with appropriate medications and intravenous fluids. The fluids were then followed by an intravenous bisphosphonate for the high calcium level. The fluids continued to be used after this but when Mrs Smith's intravenous cannula extravasated, the fluids were placed subcutaneously. They were reviewed regularly but Mrs Smith seemed less muddled and certainly less dehydrated. Her oral intake was minimal. However, despite treating the hypercalcaemia, the blood calcium levels did not decrease significantly. When Mrs Smith was in the terminal phase (only days or hours left to live) she became very chesty and her son became concerned about the noise her breathing was making. He was concerned that his mother was suffering. The nurses explained to him the cause of the chestiness, and that her body was no longer able to cope with the subcutaneous fluids. Instead of circulating them through the cardiovascular system and being filtered through the kidneys, the fluid was accumulating in her lungs. They advised that the fluids be stopped and that they would be able to administer some medication through a syringe driver which may prevent this worsening. They were quick to reassure Mrs Smith's son that Mrs Smith looked very comfortable: she was not showing any nonverbal signs of discomfort and the sound of the breathing was worse for her son than for her. The fluids were stopped, her son was pleased to note that she appeared to remain comfortable, and the syringe driver was given alongside a loading dose of the medication to prevent the secretions worsening. She died peacefully 18 hours later.

It can be seen that there were several good reasons to start Mrs Smith's fluids, and particularly so to give the intravenous bisphosphonates: she was hypercalcaemic which was causing nausea, confusion and constipation; she was dehydrated and she was unable to take enough oral fluids to help this. The fluids were continued as for only as long as they were felt to be necessary. When the side effects of the subcutaneous fluids started, that is, the terminal secretions, the fluids were stopped appropriately and Mrs Smith's son was given the necessary rationale behind this so that he understood why this was done.

Although this book is not necessarily about artificial hydration and symptom control, it is an important issue which needs addressing in terms of supportive treatment for terminally ill patients. Remember, although certain arguments and thoughts may differ from the more accepted ones, they are certainly still worth bearing in mind. This issue is one of many which have arguments for and against certain interventions, and there may be no right or wrong way to deal with it. However, if a patient begins to develop terminal secretions, the use of artificial hydration will probably make this worse and this is a good reason to stop the fluids, or not to start them in the first instance, and to use appropriate medications to prevent this worsening. A good way to explain this to family carers is to say that the cardiovascular system is not coping with the extra fluids and is causing them to accumulate on the lungs, causing noisy breathing. It is therefore best to stop these fluids and use medications in order to try and control the secretions.

It is important to remember that this may be the first time the family carers have watched a loved one die. It is very easy to wear the cloak of professionalism and give advice, but remember it may be very difficult for the family carers to appreciate this immediately. They will probably feel very guilty about any fluids and nutrition being reduced or stopped, and they will need extra support in order to realise that this is not how they need to feel and that reducing or stopping fluids or nutrition is needed in order to achieve good patient comfort. Always use sensitive words and phrases, allow time for questions and then give support. Most of all, be available. For the majority of family carers such a situation will equate to being told bad news, and thus information should be given in the way that any other bad news would be given, according to the recommendations made later on in this book.

Smith (2004) states that if death is seen as a failure rather than as an important part of life, individuals are not given the chance to prepare for it and medicine does not give the attention it should to helping people to die a 'good death'. Death has become medicalised and most people today in the UK will die in hospital, even though they may say they would prefer to die at home. Smith (2004) states that several people, including Dame Cicely Saunders, have pioneered palliative care and it is a paradox that something that happens to all of us (i.e. death) needs a speciality.

This paradox is recognised in the resuscitation guidelines (BMA *et al.*, 2001), which state:

> The primary goal of medicine is to benefit patients by restoring or maintaining their health as far as possible, thereby maximising the benefit and minimising the harm. If treatment fails, or ceases to give net benefit to the patient, or if an adult patient has competently refused the treatment, this goal cannot be realised and the justification for providing this treatment is removed. It is not an appropriate goal . . . to prolong life at all costs with no regard to its quality or the burdens of treatment on the patient.

This statement recommends that resuscitation can never be appropriate for someone in the terminal phases of illness. If Mrs Smith had been resuscitated at the point that her heart had stopped, it would not have been successful or appropriate, would have caused her son great distress and would have been distressing for the nurses and any other patients within the vicinity. Her death would not have been peaceful, dignified or 'good'.

However, the dilemma of CPR in palliative care comes for those patients who feel they have a good quality of life, remain fairly well and independent, and whom have metastatic disease. What should have been done if Mrs Smith was 30 instead of 80? The author argues that age should not come into the equation, since in Mrs Smith's situation her age was not the issue. She was very weak and was deteriorating slowly: when her heart stopped, if she had been only 30 years old, how advanced must the disease have been, or what else was going on in her body, in order for the healthy heart of a such a young woman to stop? CPR would more than likely be unsuccessful in such situations. Chapter 3 will discuss success rates of resuscitation in more detail.

Most people may think dying at home would be their choice; however, 60% of all deaths occur in hospital (Costello, 2004). Hospital resources are well used by most palliative patients in their last year of life, and 10–50% of hospital beds at any one time may be used by patients with advanced disease (Faull and Woof, 2002). Thus hospitals need to be able to provide general and specialist palliative care for such patients and their family carers. All large district and general hospitals will have their own hospital palliative care team for this purpose, but each team can only help if it actually receives the referral once the patient needs their input. Many healthcare staff may not refer patients to the palliative care team, for varying reasons: perhaps they feel they are doing a good job themselves; perhaps the family carers or patient refuse the input from the palliative care team fearing that this means they are dying; perhaps healthcare staff forget or even do not realise that the team is available for this purpose; or perhaps the staff feel nothing else can be offered and the patient is a hopeless case. Many patients slip through the net and do not receive the expert care they require and are entitled to. However good or experienced a consultant or nurse is at looking after such a patient, the expertise of the palliative care team can ensure good multi-disciplinary teamworking whilst reassuring any anxious patients and family carers that the team's input can benefit them. The palliative care team may also be able to expedite a rapid discharge for terminally ill patients to their own home if this is a possibility, or attempt to transfer them to the local hospice for more consistent specialist care.

It is easy to criticise the level of care that some dying patients may receive. However, hospitals have been built to cater for all types of illnesses, disease and trauma, not just for palliative patients. Nurses often need a tremendous amount of knowledge, not only of anatomy, physiology and hospital routine, but also of relatively new medical advances which may be used and of drug side-effects. Bearing this in mind, in the present NHS climate it may be surprising that any patients receive good nursing care. But many nurses and doctors are very committed to providing the best care they can to all patients, especially to those who are dying and their family carers. These healthcare professionals are often undervalued, yet they continue to strive for high standards of patient care in an age of strained NHS resources and time.

The hospital palliative care team works within the hospital setting while using the principles of palliative care and of the hospice movement. Dame Cecily Saunders pioneered the hospice movement in order to allow existing institutions to offer specialist palliative care. Hospital palliative care teams apply the same principles in the hospital setting, but doing this is more difficult because of staff shortages, lack of equipment and other resources, and inexperienced staff. Also, an acute hospital has been set up to provide acute care: thus the focus of palliative care will not be its forte. The most important aspect of specialist palliative care is individualised patient care. Dame Cecily's quote, in 1970, 'You matter because you are you, we will help you live until you die,' identifies the focus of the care given: it is led according to the patient's need and not according to institutional routine. There is also support for family carers and the active involvement of appropriate members of the multidisciplinary team in order to aim to achieve true holistic patient care. If Mrs Smith had felt she wanted to stay in the hospital because she had received

good care, knew the nurses well and was now too weak to go home, the intro-
duction of the hospital palliative care team to her and her son would have
allowed extra support to both of them, as well as specialist symptom control
guidance for both Mrs Smith and the ward staff and doctors.

Good palliative care can reassure patient and carers that, despite a decision
being made against having CPR and even perhaps active treatment, a good
death can be achieved. However, care of dying patients demands qualities of
a medical practitioner that do not sit neatly within the prevailing medical paradigm (Barbato, 2003). Thus death is often medicalised, and patients continue
to endure often unnecessary interventions such as blood tests and routine
monitoring of observations.

A relatively recent example of good palliative care practice is the development of the Liverpool 'Care of the Dying' pathway (Ellershaw and Wilkinson,
2003), an integrated care pathway designed to advise all involved members of
the multi-disciplinary team how to care for a terminally ill patient. It includes
information about which drugs to use for which symptoms, making sure the
patient has a DNAR decision documented and that the family is aware of the
patient's present health status. Mrs Smith could have had the care pathway
used to guide the ward staff who cared for her during the last few days of her
life, whether in the hospital, hospice, nursing home or home setting. Guidance
for symptom control support, as well as emotional and psychological support
for Mrs Smith and her son would have also been identified by the pathway.

Dying patients should receive not only good physical care but good psychological and emotional support for themselves and their family carers. Field
(1989) points out that caring for the family can be difficult for the ward nurses,
and the interaction between the ward nurses and the dying patient's family
carers is often seen as very difficult. As hard as this may be, all healthcare professionals have a duty to care for all patients, including palliative and dying
patients, and to ensure that good palliative care is provided (Nursing and
Midwifery Council, 2004). Indeed, the culture of a hospital, and its institutional
patterns of behaviour, may actually control how nurses and doctors act with
dying patients (Costello, 2004). American sociologists Glaser and Strauss
(1965) first termed the phrase the 'dying trajectory', which they used to
describe the passage of a dying patient through the various investigations and
treatments that constitute medical treatment and nursing care. A patient's
death trajectory is a perceived entity and does not have objective reality.
However, certain real events that happen along this trajectory Glaser and
Strauss termed as 'critical junctures'. Certain junctures may include being told
about a terminal diagnosis, whether a patient has any control over their hospital treatment and whether the patient's illness is likely to respond to palliative medical treatment. A patient's dying trajectory will nowadays be
increasingly individual, and many patients may have faced numerous
chemotherapy and radiotherapy treatments, only to find that they are find they
are now dying despite these interventions.

Remember that each patient journey, or death trajectory, in illness and disease will be an individual experience and the treatment and response to it (physical, emotional, psychological, financial, social and spiritual) will also be individual. Resuscitation is an important part of any patient's care and, like all medical interventions, will not always be successful in certain patients. If resuscitation decisions are faced appropriately and the correct decision made they can prevent a lot of anger, distress and the inappropriate use of limited resources.

With many new medicines and treatments becoming available in the past 50 years, advancements have been made which have helped people to live longer, successfully, but which also help people to live longer when this may mean a poor quality of life (Field, 1994). Diseases that people died from years ago such as heart disease are now able to be treated as chronic for decades: the treatment of these conditions makes them fit into a *cure* model rather then a *care* model (Neuberger, 2003). Years ago, these treatments were not available and so patient care focused more on psychological support and comfort to the dying, rather than on trying to reverse death. More appropriate care in such situations would be to withdraw inappropriate treatments and not to offer those deemed to be futile (Barbato, 2003).

Neuberger (2003) and Field (1994) argue that the hospice movement has been well accepted for many years, but it remains unacceptable to many healthcare professionals and the public, and there still remains much medicalisation of death, with doctors taking the dominant role in leading the care of those who are dying, which is often inappropriate.

THE MEDICALISATION OF DEATH

The medicalisation of illness and death means that most people will make the healthcare system their main focus of support when they are ill, reducing the importance of the family and community care to that person. Patients take on a whole new set of rules, beliefs and values whilst they are ill. Although a big focus of patient care is to try to keep patients in the community, lack of money and resources means that they often end up in hospital. The majority of deaths occur in hospital, as stated before. Hospitals often originated from workhouses and many older people feared admission into one, in case they would not come out again. Hospitals were designed to care for people with conditions that should be able to be treated. The advancement of medical technology often means people live longer with incurable illness or disease but do not have a good quality of life, or are unable to have the care they need at home and thus need to be admitted into somewhere able to give them full-time care, such as a residential or nursing home, or community hospital. Before the NHS was founded, hospitals were places with strict rules and regulations, for people who were more objects of charity rather than ill. With the advent of the NHS in

1948, the focus was on high quality care for all, irrespective of means or medical condition. However, more and more financial pressures alongside medical advancement means that needs are often put after money, with resources being cut or not extended as they should be. Lack of community care has caused bed pressures within hospitals. However, hospitals are seen as somewhere where people can die.

Patients are frequently expected by hospital staff to comply with all treatment prescribed and to be kind and 'good' patients. Those who do not comply or who question the care they are given are often labelled as 'bad' patients. Some of the patterns of care in any institution require patients to go along with the care given, to relinquish their questioning skills and power of reason, and to comply; this applies to hospitals as well.

This appears to be happening because of the merger between mainstream acute care and palliative care, where the experience of suffering is now re-characterised as a medical problem with a solution. The medicalisation of death can be seen as the expansion of what, in medicine, is seen as relevant to the good practice of life (Field, 1994). Palliative care has emerged because of the over-medicalisation of death, and to manage distressing symptoms (Costello, 2004). Illich (1990) argues that death has been seen as less of an inevitable part of life and more of a failure. He described the medicalisation of dying as a loss of the capacity to accept death and suffering as meaningful aspects of life; there is a sense of being in a state of 'total war' against death at all stages of the life cycle. There is also a crippling of personal and family care and a devaluing of traditional rituals which previously surrounded death and dying, and the medicalisation of death forms a social control in which a rejection of 'patient-hood' by dying or bereaved people is labelled as a form of deviance. Field (1994) states that death is no longer seen as an acceptable part of life in the way that it was before the industrial and medical revolutions. He also argues that family responsibilities are less clear-cut now, with increasing separations and divorces, and so the responsibility for the dying tends now to be taken over by, and is expected to be provided by, the state. Hospital deaths have increased in numbers over home deaths because of this.

Costello (2004) argues that the advent of palliative care medicine and nursing care in the late 1980s has been viewed by some as to be further medicalization of death, not as preventing it. Many palliative patients are living longer, requiring extended care because their lifespan is being elongated through palliative medical treatments. Also, many of the care decisions which traditionally would have been made by the family are now being made by the patient or the medical team. Having the patient die in a hospital or hospice, surrounded by doctors and healthcare staff, rather than by their family carers, and by making private something which used to be shared publicly by the local community, can be interpreted as the medicalisation of death. Costello (2004) also argues that the use of certain drugs to control symptoms may also be seen as the medicalisation of death. Even a DNAR order made by medical staff could be seen as a loss of control by patients or their family carers, however appropriate they realise the decision is. Costello (2004) continues that the dying trajectory, as defined by Glaser and Strauss (1965), is easily influenced by the biomedical model of care, and can lead to the disempowerment of patients either by making decisions about care in hospital, or from other influences of medical care at hospital and at home.

However with the advent of palliative care in the 1980s there has been an increase in the number of support roles available for those dying at home, in hospital or in the hospice. But the lack of finances means that many of these posts and resources are funded by charities, such as the hospice movement, the Macmillan cancer relief charity and the Marie Curie charity. Society and medicine are accepting palliative care more readily, but the state is not able, or willing, to provide what is needed to allow a 'good' death for terminally ill patients.

WHAT IS A 'GOOD' DEATH?

What constitutes a 'good' death? It has been given different interpretations, such as the actual moment of death itself, as in euthanasia, or to an acceptable approach to death and dying. It can, however, be a set of relations and preparations: not just a single event but a series of social events (McNamara *et al.*, 1994). Many studies have looked into this but, needless to say, there are stages involved in acceptance of the dying process and these have been influenced by the work of Kubler-Ross (1969), on the stages of grief and bereavement.

The Debate of the Age, Health and Care Study Group (1999) and Holland (2003) outline the principles of a good death:

- To know when death is coming and to understand what can be expected.
- To be afforded dignity and privacy.
- To have control over pain relief and other symptom control.
- To be able to retain control of what happens.
- To have choice and control over where death occurs.
- To have access to information and expertise of whatever kind is necessary.
- To have access to spiritual or emotional support required.
- To have access to hospice care in any location, not only in hospital.
- To have control over who is present and who shares the end.
- To be able to issue advance directives that ensure wishes are respected.
- To have time to say goodbye, and control over other aspects of timing.
- To be able to leave when it is time to go and not to have life prolonged pointlessly.

However, the focus should not all be only on the actual dying process. If discussions about death are more acceptable through becoming part of regular life, such as being included in education in schools, society can begin to accept death as part of everyday life, as it was before the industrial and medical revolutions.

What makes an expected, terminal death different from unexpected cardiac or respiratory arrest? Durham (1994) outlines how the body begins to slowly close down. During the final few hours before death, the changes to the brain and all the body's systems mean that there are often changes in breathing patterns, called Cheyne–Stokes breathing, where the breath becomes slower and shallower, stops for a short while (the apnoeic stage) then restarts much deeper and gradually becomes shallower again until another break in the breathing occurs. This is because the neural centres in the cerebrum lose control of the respiratory rhythm. A lower control centre in the medulla responds by regulating respiration solely in response to changes in blood carbon dioxide levels. During the apnoeic phase chemoreceptors in the aortic arch, carotid body and medulla fail to initiate respiration. Increased load on the heart due to lowered blood pressure and increased ventricular filling during the hyper-apnoeic phase may cause heart failure. In the dying phase the heart fails in its pumping functions, resulting in insufficient perfusion, ischaemia and cell death. The skin becomes cool to the touch and may appear mottled or blue, the pulse becomes weaker and thready. Renal output lessens or stops because of the reduced cardiac output. Reduced gut motility can result in faecal impaction and cause the patient to become restless. The patient needs less nutrition but will need regular mouth care to prevent discomfort, often increased by mouth breathing. Decreasing brain function may result in confusion and restlessness, apathy and lethargy, stupor, withdrawal and failure to respond to normal stimuli. There may be emotional changes, such as fear of dying, unusual behaviour such as plucking at the bedclothes, or inappropriate laughing or verbal responses. Pain may be experienced even though any pain existing before this time may have been well-controlled. If the patient cannot explain this verbally non-verbal signs often include frowning, taut facial muscles and stiffening of the body muscles when moved. It is important to maintain or increase analgesics at this stage: these should not be withdrawn without good reason. This shows how dying affects all of the body's systems, not just the cardiac and respiratory systems.

The experience of death lives on with the relatives and carers of patients long after they have died, and thus a good death, where the patient is physically and psychologically comfortable, can provide many good memories for the family, reassuring them that their relative did not suffer unnecessarily. Field (1994) says a good death includes effective communication between the patient, the family and healthcare workers, involving them in decisions and explaining the rationale behind all the care and treatments given. Palgi and Abramovitch (1984) link the concept of a good death to the hospice movement, which was developed to prevent the depersonalisation of death often seen in hospital care. The hospice, and palliative care, focuses on the physical, psychological, spiritual and social needs of patients and their carers

(McNamara *et al.*, 1994; McNeil, 1998), caring for patients and their family carers as part of a social unit, not as an individual. A good death involves acceptance by patients and their carers that death will happen soon, and involves good physical care for patients in order to meet any symptom control needs during this period. It also involves patients being where they want to be when they die where possible (McNeil, 1998). The medicalisation of death is not viewed as a 'good' death since many doctors are not knowledgeable about the approaches and principles used in palliative care.

In order for there to be acceptance of approaching death, Poss (1981) argues that there are six tasks that need to be completed.

- An awareness of impending death: to be given by the use of proper words, not euphemisms.
- Hope and fear: there is to be a balance between the two. Hope that the person will be spared unnecessary suffering, but fear that they must be realistic about death. Where hope is absent, fear takes over.
- An active decision to reverse the physical survival processes: there is a voluntary relinquishment of the will to live.
- Relinquishing responsibility and independence: there is submission to the situation, and acceptance.
- Separation and disengagement (from life itself): letting others take over certain life roles which the patient, once carried out themself.
- Spiritual preparation: for the future 'afterlife', whatever form it takes for the patients. It can be faith-based or not.

Who decides if what the patient, and their family carers, experienced was a good death? Healthcare professionals have defined it as controlling physical symptoms and psychologically preparing the patient for death, whereas a bad death is when physical symptoms are not controlled and psychological distress is not faced (Low and Payne, 1996).

Healthcare professionals can actually contribute to ensuring a dying person and their family carers experience a good death, according to Neuberger (2004). The dying process itself can be enhanced by those caring for the patient, be it healthcare professionals or family carers, if the patient is well supported and listened to. Part of achieving a good death comes from caring for the family carers and friends of patients as well. How the family carers view the death will have a huge influence on their grieving process. One important thing stated by Neuberger (2004) is that healthcare professionals need to try and prevent an atmosphere of dishonesty that can often occur between couples or family carers and friends when someone they know is dying. Often this comes about because they fear that honesty may cause distress. This means that many things that need to be discussed with the patient, such as a will or certain things that need to be said to various other people, do not occur and this can actually result in the patient's death not being viewed as a good death. Healthcare professionals need to be prepared for patients who may want to talk about their death, be it imminent or not, and that this may cause distress to the family carers. This will mean that their personal view of death and dying, and even their view of their own mortality, must be faced honestly.

Neuberger (2004) outlines other issues which can influence a good death. These include being aware of the person's cultural and religious beliefs in order not to cause offence; asserting professional leadership in order to resolve any previous conflicts which may have arisen in decision-making, when patients can no longer make their own choices; having some knowledge of the psychology of grief and thus recognising why certain people may react in different ways at the time of the patient's death; and the use of empathy. Knowing what *not* to say is more important than worrying about *what* to say. Words cannot always help, in which case it is acceptable for the healthcare professional not to say anything.

Neuberger (2004) gives a very good account of what is seen as a 'good' death, in her book, *Dying Well*. She states that attitudes to death are confirmed by the euphemisms for the word *death* that Western society tends to use. Instead of saying that someone has died, phrases such as 'passed away' or 'fell asleep' may be used instead. Other less sensitive ones include 'popped their clogs' or 'turned their toes up'. There seems to be a real embarrassment of how death is perceived, judging by some of the phrases used. These euphemisms seem to have really come into use in England only since the end of the Victorian era. This seems strange when death at that time was a normal, frequent occurrence. In fact, the Victorians upstaged dealing with grief and bereavement by wearing black clothes (after Queen Victoria wore black following the death of Prince Albert) and paying more attention to the funeral and wake. Great pride was taken in how the funeral was conducted and until recently many people put a regular amount of money aside to pay for their funeral. Neuberger (2004) maintains that death became something very unfashionable in the 1970s and 1980s, mainly because of attitudes to death from the first and second world wars, in which many soldiers and civilians were killed. Around the beginning of the twentieth century the development of communications coincided with the First World War, and this meant that many people heard about the death of a relative more quickly than they would have done previously. Nowadays, Neuberger (2004) states, death is almost fashionable again and the upsurge of the hospice movement and specialist palliative care services has helped this. However, death is still often dealt with in an unemotional and practical way.

Jacqueline Clark (2003) says that healthcare professionals should focus on the patient's concepts of a good death, not just what the professionals feel is a good death. She feels more research should be carried out into what this may include, and it should not just concentrate on physical symptoms or statistics stating what the patient finally died of.

David Clark (2002) describes the main elements of a good death in Western medicine:

- pain-free
- open acknowledgement of the imminence of death
- death at home, surrounded by friends and family
- an 'aware' death, in which personal conflicts and unfinished business are resolved
- death as a personal growth
- death according to personal preference and in a manner that resonates with the person's individuality.

So when does a patient come under the blanket of palliative care? It seems at first that cancer care comes under the convenient categories of curative, palliative and terminal. However, 'cure' may mean different things to different people. Doctors may talk in terms of five-year survival, when patients tend to be discharged from follow-up clinics and technically seen as cured, whereas patients may see 'cure' in terms of definite survival from the cancer until another cause of death occurs, usually in many years time. Sepulveda *et al.* (2002) define palliative care as:

> An approach that improves quality of life of patients and their families facing the problems associated with life-threatening illness, through prevention and relief of suffering by means of early identification and impeccable assessment and treatment of pain and other problems, physical, psychosocial and spiritual.

In the context of the principles of palliative care from the World Health Organization (WHO, 2002, p. 14) these same principles can be applied in curative illness as well, which can be termed as 'supportive' care rather then palliative (NICE, 2004). Even palliative care patients may still be offered chemotherapy or radiotherapy: treatments which many patients may think are only curative, to control their disease. Thus palliative care principles can be applied in many situations, and should be applied when caring for any adult patient. However, for the purpose of this book, CPR will focus only on those patients who have incurable diseases.

The NCPC (2002b) differentiates between *general* palliative care, which can be offered by all healthcare professionals for low to medium complex patient problems, and *specialist* palliative care services, for patients with complex palliative problems. Specialist palliative care includes hospice support, community Macmillan support, palliative care nurse specialist and consultants' support and Marie Curie nursing. However, such resources are being used increasingly for patients with low to medium complexity problems as there are few practitioners able to offer this care within the hospital and community because of lack of staff and resources.

Harrold (2002) argues that sometimes it is not clear if someone is dying until death is imminent. The disease process may have taken over much more quickly than anticipated, even for patients in remission, and even then someone may be described as 'dying' but may well survive through the episode and live longer. Alternatively, she argues, others may live a frail life and die without a period called 'dying' having been identified. This ambiguity makes coping with and planning for death very difficult, especially if coping and planning are based on being sure that someone is dying, being sure that treatments are no longer effective and being sure that patients' wishes and choices are being honoured. It may be possible to use any 'false alarms' to produce some advance care planning (Harrold, 2002) when any arrangements that had not been previously discussed will be faced and plans made, such as place of death, any funeral arrangements and sorting out a will. However, flexibility with any plans is needed in case feelings change when the inevitable happens.

Harrold (2002) continues that there is no medical definition of someone being 'terminally ill' and that, in fact, many people may live with a terminal illness for a long time before they die. Estimating prognosis may people help but Harrold (2002) continues that this is often very inaccurate, with one study showing that patients given a prognosis within 24 hours before they died were given a 10% chance of living for six months (Lynn *et al.*, 1997). The outcome of this ambiguity is to support patients and carers as much as possible, and not to assume that what is happening to the patient is irreversible; and being as honest as possible with patients and family carers.

Death need not be medicalised, however difficult facing it may be, not only for patients and their family carers, but also for healthcare professionals. A good death requires discussion and planning. Although this can be distressing for some, a good death can leave better memories for those left behind.

3 Resuscitation guidelines, success and futility, and medical paternalism

As stated in the previous chapters the British Medical Association, Royal College of Nursing and the Resuscitation Council (UK) have produced guidelines on resuscitation (BMA *et al.*, 2001, first published 1993). It is still evident that many healthcare personnel are not aware of these guidelines, including trained nurses (Bass, 2003). However, they are recommended as a basis for all local cardiopulmonary resuscitation (CPR) trust policies and guidelines. It is imperative that all healthcare professionals are aware of and have at least a basic understanding of the guidelines.

The purpose of the resuscitation guidelines is to identify the key ethical and legal principles that should underpin all resuscitation decisions. These basic principles apply to all patients in all settings, but because a wide range of clinical and personal matters have to be taken into account for each patient, each resuscitation decision will be an individual one.

It is important for every healthcare professional to read not only their local resuscitation policy but also to read the actual resuscitation guidelines (BMA *et al.*, 2001). This whole document was recommended to National Health Service (NHS) Trusts in September 2000 by an NHS circular in which the chief executives of all the trusts were required to ensure that appropriate resuscitation policies, which respect patients' wishes, were in place, were understood by all relevant staff and accessible to those who needed them, as well being as subject to audit and monitoring.

THE SUCCESS AND FUTILTY OF CPR

As noted in Chapter 1, resuscitation is not always appropriate for every person, and it can be futile. What is meant by 'futile'? Definitions include:

- When treatment offers no benefit to the patient because maximal therapy has failed and physiologic improvement is impossible. (Lo, 1991)

- When important goals of care cannot be achieved, although other goals might be. (LeVack, 2002)
- If reasoning and experience indicate that the intervention would be highly unlikely to result in a meaningful survival for that patient. (American Thoracic Society, 1991)

Thus in the case of Mrs Smith (see Case Study 1) resuscitation was not offered because it was not expected to be successful: her heart and breathing stopped because of a terminal event, caused by her terminal cancer.

Rousseau (2000) adds that an action is futile when it causes needless pain and suffering, and when it will not achieve the goal of restoring the patient to an acceptable quality of life. He continues that in order for doctors to decide if an intervention will be futile or not, they need to ask themselves four questions:

- Will the intervention provide benefit to the patient (the ethical principle of beneficence)?
- Will the intervention cause greater harm than good (the ethical principle of non-maleficence)?
- What is the patient's preference (or what do the family carers feel the patient's preference would be)?
- What physical, social and financial costs will the intervention involve (the ethical principle of justice)?

Patients or their family carers may request futile interventions for several reasons, including feelings of guilt towards the patient, or because they have unrealistic goals and beliefs about what the intervention will achieve. Perhaps they mistrust doctors because of past experiences, or are a different social class from the doctors, or perhaps are even denying that the patient is dying. They may have difficulty in communicating due to a different language, culture and beliefs. Honesty at this point should help to alleviate most of these concerns and unrealistic demands. Doctors are not obliged to provide a futile treatment, even if the patient or family carers demand it. If explaining why resuscitation is not appropriate does not assist the patient or family carers to fully understand, it may be appropriate for a doctor to refer the patient to another doctor for a second opinion. Although this may seem a waste of limited time healthcare professionals should understand they are dealing with inexperienced people who risk losing someone they love or who risk losing their own life. What seems obvious to someone involved in a caring profession may not be clear to patients and their family carers. Having a second opinion, even when it may not differ, may enable patients and family carers to cope better psychologically with Do Not Attempt Resuscitation (DNAR) decisions, and with approaching death.

It is important to remember that what seems futile to a doctor or other healthcare professionals may actually help to relieve the patient psychologically; for example oxygen therapy which may not be needed accord-ing to oxygen saturation levels but which may make the patient feel they can breathe more easily. Such small interventions can reassure patients that they are receiving good care, and may allow them to have a small amount of choice in a situation they feel totally without control and totally beholden to. However, this does not mean that attempting CPR will also help.

Wilkinson (2002) argues that there *is* an obvious reason for not providing harmful treatments, but the basis for *not* providing futile treatments is less obvious. He argues that the BMA has stated that healthcare professionals are not obliged to provide any treatment which cannot produce the desired effect. 'Harm' deals with treatments where the burdens outweigh the benefits, whereas 'futile' describes treatments that will almost certainly not produce the desired benefit. Wilkinson (2002) continues to argue that not offering treat-ment just because it is futile is not really enough. He states that the main reasons for not offering treatment are:

- the treatment in question is harmful to the patient: if so, it is not merely futile
- the treatment in question does not constitute an effective use of healthcare resources
- quality of life for the patient is so bad, for example the patient is uncon-scious and suffering intractable pain or distress, that choosing non-treatment rather than treatment will benefit them by allowing them to die.

From this argument it may be argued that a DNAR decision in terminal illness would be appropriate since it would prevent resuscitation taking place, which would be harmful to the patient; it would have more side effects than bene-fits, such as fracturing ribs and causing neurological damage, and the patient's quality of life at such a stage is very poor.

Wilkinson (2002) concludes by arguing that any withdrawal of treatment for reasons not listed above would be ethically controversial and regarded by some as a form of euthanasia.

LeVack (2002), however, does warn about the concept of futility by saying:

What about the concept of futility? The way in which we make decisions deter-mines the choices we give patients and there is no doubt that doctors do make value judgements. They have always done so. If, however, they have to be influ-enced by the patient's own values does futility, as a concept, help them understand them? I think not.

So, how futile is resuscitation in palliative patients? Successful resuscitation rates have increased due to modern technology, the advent of coronary care units, better more accessible resuscitation training and the establishment of expert bodies for advice and guidance, such as the UK and European Resus-citation Councils (Hayward, 1999). (There are now many resuscitation coun-cils worldwide.) These success rates have particularly increased in coronary

care units compared to general wards with initial survival following resuscitation at almost 50%, and with one-year survival of nearly 20%. Compare this
with general wards where survival after one year is 11% (Tunstall-Pedoe
et al., 1992). However, Bains (1998) and Ewer et al. (2001) feel that resuscitation success is now decreasing because increasing attempts are being made to
raise the dead and dying, rather than revive the living.

Hayward (1999) poses the question, though, of what constitutes success?
Factors which should be included in success are long-term survival, quality of
life after the resuscitation and any neurological damage sustained from the
resuscitation itself. If not outlined in detail in any resuscitation research, such
factors may make the issues of *success*, which have been quoted in resuscitation, contentious and subjective.

Healthcare professionals' views of resuscitation success are often unrealistic and overoptimistic (Miller et al., 1993; Ghusan et al., 1995; Wagg et al., 1995)
and the public's views are often skewed by the media (Diem et al., 1996). High
profile stories have increased the public's awareness of resuscitation and
DNAR orders (Mendrick and Dillon, 2000). Survival to discharge from hospital, after cardiac arrest has been quoted at different rates, and what needs
to be taken into account in palliative care is that many of these statistics may
not include details of primary or secondary cancer. For instance, patients with
primary breast or prostate cancer and secondary bone disease may have a
better prognosis than those with a lung primary and secondary bone disease.
This is important since not all patients with metastatic cancer have as poor a
prognosis as others. Table 3.1 lists some of the resuscitation success rates available in the literature. The statistics that have been specified for cancer patients
are marked.

Table 3.1 includes the work of Ewer et al. (2001) which uses a clear explanation of how to differentiate between patients who are in the terminal stages
of their disease, that is, anticipated cardiac arrest, and those who are not, that
is, unanticipated cardiac arrest. This may be a way for healthcare professionals to feel more supported and able to substantiate those patients who should
be for resuscitation and which should not.

The work of Vitelli et al. (1991) stated that the research they carried out was
on cancer patients over a three-year period. Their opening sentence states that:
'Cardiac arrest in a cancer patient is commonly accepted as a terminal event'.
They continue that less than 50% of patients who survive being resuscitated
in hospital will survive to discharge, and less than 20% will survive long enough
to leave the hospital alive following resuscitation.

It is not difficult to realise by looking at Table 3.1 that there is quite a difference in the success rates quoted for CPR, even for research where cancer
statistics may not be included. There is, however, less chance of being discharged from hospital after resuscitation than there is of initial success.

Some of the research quoted in Table 3.1 does not specify certain important
factors which could sway the success of resuscitation: where the arrest took

Table 3.1 Comparison of quoted success rates of studies on CPR

Reference	On cancer patients?	Year	Survival: initial success rate (%)	Survival to discharge (%)
Vitelli *et al.*	Yes	1991	65.7	10.5
Varon *et al.*	Yes	1998		9.6
Myatra, *et al.*	Yes	2004		22.4
Wallace *et al.*	Yes	2002		2
Ewer *et al.*	Yes	2001		0–2 (in anticipated)
				22.2 (in unanticipated)
Ebell *et al.*	Not stated	1998	41	13
McGrath	Not stated	1987	53	15
Wallace *et al.*	Not stated	2002		0–22
Karetsky *et al.*	Not stated	1995		3–21
Faber-Langendoen (review of nine CPR studies)	Not stated	1991		
Kouwenhoven *et al.*	No	1960		70
Murphy *et al.*	Not stated	1989	83	6.5
Hollingsworth	Not stated	1969		
Johnson *et al.*	Not stated	1967		
Camarata *et al.*	Not stated	1971		
Lemire and Johnson	Not stated	1972		
Messert and Quaglieri	Not stated	1976		
Peatfield *et al.*	Not stated	1977		
Fusagen and Summa	Not stated	1978		5–23
DeBard	Not stated	1981		
Scott	Not stated	1981		
Hershy and Fisher	Not stated	1982		
Bedell *et al.*	Not stated	1984		
Gulati *et al.*	Not stated	1983		
Castagna and Shubin	Not stated	1974		

place (e.g. coronary care unit, ITU or general ward); whether the survivors experienced any post-arrest complications and whether these were long-lasting effects; where the survivors were discharged to; the quality of life of patients pre- and post-arrest and resuscitation; and whether those who survived, or did not, had pre-existing co-morbid factors which may have decreased resuscitation success (Broadway *et al.*, 1993). There is also no mention of certain influencing factors such as which healthcare professionals were involved and what their own experience of resuscitation was, or how long had passed between the actual arrest and the start of the resuscitation. For research on cancer patients (apart from that by Ewer *et al.*, 2001) it is not specific where the primary cancer was, how many had metastatic disease and whether the arrest was due a possible terminal event.

RESUSCITATION IN A HOSPICE

Successful resuscitation is much more likely in the hospital setting than a hospice (Farsides, 2003; Dallain, 2004) as in the acute setting there are resuscitation teams and resources nearby. In a hospice, CPR necessitates calling an ambulance and a transfer to the acute hospital setting. Due to the nature of hospice care it is anticipated that few patients cared for there will be appropriate for resuscitation. With the advent of the 'Right to Life' section within the Human Rights Act of 1998 a blanket DNAR policy is no longer acceptable within any institution and is considered unethical. Most patients in a hospice would be seen as inappropriate to resuscitate on the grounds of medical futility. However, as hospices increasingly now take non-malignant cases, or those reviewed in the outpatients or day services for symptom control but having curative treatment, some of these patients may be appropriate for resuscitation. These individuals should be given the choice of opting-in for resuscitation, a decision which should be discussed with them and then regularly re-assessed. Every hospice should have a resuscitation policy, and information concerning CPR should be readily available for patients and their family carers.

Following on from this, the NCPC (2003) states that patients admitted to a hospice must be aware of the hospice philosophy of care, which tends to be that active treatment for patients, rather than resuscitation, is the norm. Staff, inpatients and day centre patients must be informed about this, and patients may be given the opportunity to 'opt in' for resuscitation, especially if their disease is not advanced.

So, 'Lies, damn lies and statistics' (Benjamin Disraeli) can be clearly seen to apply here. Statistics can say almost whatever researchers want to emphasise. However, Table 3.1 does show a relatively lower success rate for research specifically involving cancer patients.

There are three main predictors of survival after CPR:

- whether the arrest was witnessed
- whether basic life support is commenced quickly
- whether defibrillation is carried out as early as possible in cases of ventricular fibrillation, and pulseless ventricular tachycardia (Ballew, 1997).

As well as these predictors, Birtwhistle and Nielson (1998) found evidence of certain prognostic indicators which can decrease the success of resuscitation. These include renal failure, cancer pneumonia, sepsis, hypotension and patients aged 60 years or more (Rozenbaum and Shenkman, 1988; O'Keefe et al., 1991; Ebell, 1992; Cohn et al., 1993; Schultz et al., 1996). Age has previously been seen as a factor to consider when deciding someone's resuscitation status. Obviously the human body becomes less strong with age but this differs with each individual. With the advent of the *National Service Framework for*

Older People (DoH, 2001) age discrimination should be obliterated. This framework states that NHS services will be provided, regardless of age, on the basis of clinical need alone: the failure of healthcare professionals to follow guidance on the use of DNAR orders is part of a wider concern over ageism in the NHS (Ebrahim, 2000). The concept of a 'good innings' is a thing of the past. Dimond (2002) states:

> There are, in law, no age limits for accessing treatment. The only criteria are the prognosis of the patient, and the extent to which further investment in their health is justified in terms of the benefit that it would bring to that individual.

Therefore, age alone is not enough to base a resuscitation decision on. Disease status and health are more objective and ethical bases on which to make such a decision.

George *et al.* (1989) took assessment for resuscitation success further by devising a point system whereby certain pre-existing prognostic factors are given a score. There is a score of 3 for each of the following: hypotension (systolic equal or <90 mmHg); azotaemia (blood urea equal to >17.9 mmol/L or serum creatinine equal to or >200 mmol/L); malignancy; pneumonia; and homebound lifestyle. There is a score of 1 for each of the following: angina; acute myocardial infarction; heart failure; S3 gallop; oliguria (urine output of <300 mL per day); sepsis; mechanical ventilation; recent ventilation; coma; and cirrhosis. Any patient scoring 7 is predicted only a 15% chance of survival post-arrest. A score of 8 or more indicates the patient would be unlikely to survive. It is interesting that age is not included in this assessment. But it is important to remember that it is possible for many younger people to have less success when resuscitated than older people, because of pre-existing co-morbid, possibly congenital, factors.

The disadvantage of a scoring system, such as the one devised by George *et al.* (1989) is that it is yet another piece of paper to be filled in by healthcare professionals; it does not involve talking to the patient and family carers about their choices, if there are any; it states 'malignancy' and not where the primary tumour is or whether there is metastatic disease (certain non-metastatic cancers can have a longer survival and better chance of cure or remission). However, 'Neither metastatic disease nor age (*per se*) are predictive of response to CPR' (Varon *et al.*, 1998). One possible advantage of such a point system being used in the pre-assessment of resuscitation success is that it could be used as a guide for less experienced healthcare professionals, as long as it is completed accurately.

Resuscitation is therefore not 100% successful, and inappropriate resuscitation has several consequences (Birtwhistle and Nielson, 1998):

- the person may be denied a dignified death
- it may be distressing for the family carers
- a cardiac team can become demoralised of they are always 'failing'

- other patients may be denied care or treatment while the crash team is pre-occupied with CPR
- there may be an inappropriate use of valuable resources.

The NCPC (2003) provides some broad generalisations in terms of CPR success (despite the different settings, diagnosis, the patients included, hospital sites and so on).

- *Overall* (for all patient groups, not just palliative): one in eight of those undergoing CPR in hospital will survive to discharge and one in three of those who survive CPR will subsequently be discharged.
- CPR is most effective in people with reversible medical conditions, who have a witnessed, sudden disturbance of heart rhythm in a hospital setting.
- CPR is least effective in people who suffer a non-witnessed arrest, such as outside hospital; or in those who have a co-morbid disease such as pneumonia, sepsis, heart disease, hypoxia; or where a resuscitation attempt is prolonged (*see also* O'Keefe *et al.*, 1991). Specific surveys of patients with cancer suggest that the patient's performance status (i.e. a scoring system used to assess how patients will tolerate therapy: the lower the score, the increased risk of toxicity) prior to the cardio-pulmonary–respiratory arrest, and the presence or absence of co-morbid and progressive, unresponsive medical conditions are predictive factors:
  - a patient spending 50% or more of their time in bed had a 2–3% chance of survival to discharge (Vitelli *et al.*, 1991)
  - patients with cancer suffering an unanticipated cardiac arrest had a 22% chance of survival to discharge (Ewer *et al.*, 2001)
  - a patient with cancer suffering an anticipated cardiac arrest due to pre-existing medical conditions unresponsive to treatment had a 0–2% survival rate to discharge (Ewer *et al.*, 2001; Wallace *et al.*, 2002) and thus unlikely to be successful in a patient dying from advanced, progressive disease.

Randall (for NCPC, 2003) states that if a patient is dying it is imperative to prevent unnecessary harm, and therefore to withhold CPR in this situation would be morally justified, irrespective of the patient's and family's wishes. Randall continues to argue that in other palliative care patients, particularly those who are reasonably active, who then experience a sudden, unexpected cardio-respiratory arrest, CPR may be effective, but it cannot be stated whether it will be successful; the (scant) evidence suggests CPR cannot be disregarded in such cases on the grounds of futility. This is particularly relevant given that the spectrum of patients in an inpatient unit continues to change: patients are seen earlier in their disease when they may develop reversible causes of cardiopulmonary arrest, including cardiac problems.

The resuscitation guidelines state that an advance decision not to attempt CPR should only be made after:

the appropriate consultation and consideration of all relevant aspects of the patient's condition: these include:

- The likely outcome, including likelihood of successfully restarting the patient's heart and breathing, and the overall benefit achieved from a successful resuscitation;
- The patient's known, or ascertainable, wishes;
- The patient's Human Rights, including the right to life and the right to be free from degrading treatment. (BMA *et al.*, 2001)

The resuscitation guidelines also outline circumstances where it is inappropriate to consider CPR:

- Where attempting CPR will not restart the patient's heart and breathing.
- Where there is no benefit in restarting the patient's heart and breathing. Although in most cases there is benefit gained when a patient's heart and breathing are successfully restarted following cardiopulmonary arrest, this is not true in all cases. No benefit is gained if only a very brief extension of life can be achieved and the patient's co-morbidity is such that imminent death cannot be averted.
- Where the expected benefit is outweighed by the burdens.

There are many circumstances in which it is justified to attempt to prolong life by treatment which carries side-effects, burdens and risks. Attempted CPR carries a risk of significant side-effects (such as sternal fracture, rib fracture, and splenic fracture) and most patients require either coronary care or ICU in the post-resuscitation period. A delay between cardiopulmonary arrest and resuscitation [and] the patient will suffer brain damage. Where there is a chance of good or reasonable quality of life being gained most patients willingly risk some disadvantage. The courts have confirmed it is lawful to withhold CPR on the basis that it would not confer a benefit upon the patient. (BMA *et al.*, 2001).

The NCPC (2002a) adds another reason not to attempt CPR: 'Where the competent patient refuses'.

Regnard and Randall (2005) produced a flowchart to help make advance resuscitation decisions. The chart asks three questions: first, 'Is it impossible to anticipate the particular circumstances in which CPR treatment is proposed?' If yes, then it is not possible to make an advanced decision and so CPR should be carried out unless the patient requests otherwise. If no, go to the second question: 'Is the team certain as it can be that CPR treatment could help the patient?' If yes, this is an anticipated cardio-respiratory arrest and is likely to occur due to reversible condition. In this situation they advise an advance statement and decision on CPR is possible but should be discussed with the patient to see if they have any views on this. If an arrest occurs, CPR actions should be taken according to the patient's wishes. If no, go to the next question: 'Is the team as certain as it can be that CPR treatment cannot help the patient?' If yes, it is likely the patient will die of an irreversible condition and therefore should not be for CPR. A DNAR order should be signed and communicated to those caring for the patient. The patient or family carers may be told they are not for resuscitation and the rationale as to why explained.

Willard (2000) states that there may be a place for resuscitation in palliative care, although the two seem incompatible because they have different intentions. However, resuscitation is considered acceptable by the NCPC and the Association of Palliative Medicine (APM) if it would result in a quality of life acceptable to the patient. The resuscitation decision must also require a comprehensive assessment of the patient's views and values and why they may believe that they have an acceptable quality of life. Thus, personal values may challenge science, and challenge is something many healthcare professionals are not comfortable with. Patient autonomy should also be taken into account, to buttress medical paternalism and to show it is important to value patients' life, choice and views. Patient autonomy seems to be even more significant when a person has a short lifespan, in order to allow as much patient choice as possible, and give some chances of control in an increasingly uncontrollable situation. Assisting the patient to define and achieve goals and integrate meaning, even when dying, is actually part of the process of attempting to improve quality of life, and represents the desire to respect autonomy. Quality of life is a subjective thing and can only be measured accurately by patients themselves. Thus healthcare professionals, if they want to uphold patient autonomy, should discuss resuscitation decisions with patients.

Willard (2002) goes on to argue that palliative care is concerned with the many facets of the patient's life, and is not just confined to treating physical disease. In one of the palliative care principles (as outlined in Chapter 1) death is regarded as an inevitable consequence of living. Resuscitation, however, aims to reverse this and restore life. It involves messy, invasive procedures which many would see as undignified. If resuscitation is unsuccessful, which has been seen to be more probable than not in palliative patients, it would be the antithesis of a 'good death'. There are therefore powerful arguments against resuscitation regarding quality of life and quality of death.

Regarding local CPR policies, the resuscitation guidelines state that they must include up-to-date clinical information and also that, 'Blanket policies which deny attempts at resuscitation to a group of patients, for example, to patients in a nursing home or to patients above a certain age, are unethical and probably unlawful under provisions of the Human Rights Act'. Traditionally, given that hospices originally provided terminal care, it is unsurprising that resuscitation has not been offered to hospice inpatients. In contrast, there seems to be widespread use of resuscitation in hospital, and concern that it may be indiscriminate (Willard, 2002). The resuscitation guidelines also point out that inappropriate CPR not only carries burdens for patients and their carers, but that, 'Repeated attempts at CPR which provide only short-lived clinical success can be emotionally very difficult for people close to the patient, can lower the morale and enthusiasm of the healthcare team and may mean that experienced staff and equipment are not available to attempt to resuscitate a patient for whom there is better chance of success' (BMA *et al.*, 2001; also Lo, 1991).

Once a resuscitation decision has been made for the patient, whether for or against CPR, it must be reviewed regularly in view of the patient's condition and wishes. 'Regularly' can be a very subjective concept and can very much depend on the condition of the patient. However, those who have worked with cancer patients for any length of time will be aware of how quickly a patient's condition can change, and so a more realistic review would be weekly, or sooner if the patient's condition indicates this.

Most of the public do not really understand what is entailed in resuscitation, and if the rationale behind a DNAR decision is explained most people will tend to agree with it. Who, after all, wants futile treatment, either for themselves or their close family or friends? A resuscitation decision can be a conflict of interest between the patient and doctor, when a patient with a poor prognosis may strongly request resuscitation. Tomlinson and Brody (1998) argue that a doctor could still place a DNAR order without the agreement of the patient, as the final resuscitation decision is down to the doctor in charge of that patient's care. This may, however, cause a dilemma for the nurses, who according to the National Midwifery Council *Code of Professional Conduct* (NMC, 2004) must, 'Act always in such a manner as to promote and safeguard the interests and well-being of patients and clients'. So, argues Hayward (1999) what then is the best interest of the nurse: to advocate the patients' wishes no matter how futile the chance of success, or realistically acknowledging resuscitation is inappropriate but then not being able to advocate for the patient?

Gulati (1983) controversially argues that if a patient is content with their quality of life, respect for life and patient autonomy should rule out the possibility of a DNAR order. Others have agreed with this thought (Younger, 1988; DeGross, 1990; Murphy *et al.*, 1994), that if, 'Survival is only likely to be in hours/days this, to the patient, may not be deemed futile, and they may therefore have the right to postpone death'. Stewart *et al.* (2003) continue that doctors should, 'respect patient's wishes to receive treatment which carries only a very small chance of success or benefit'. Elwell (2000) adds that upon admission to an acute hospital many patients and families have expectations of a cure, or improvement, and restoration of health. 'Anything less than the pursuit of a curative acute treatment goal may be unacceptable to them . . . In this worldview, withholding CPR is not so much an avoidance of useless treatment as an abandonment of the hope of "cure".' However, is it morally and ethically right to resuscitate someone who is likely to die shortly afterwards? (Bass, 2003). The following statement holds very true and many may agree with this more than with the previous statement: 'CPR is perceived as a definite life-saving procedure [but] it has also prolonged the process of dying and denied many patient a dignified and peaceful death' (Dean, 2001).

Despite these arguments it is only fair when looking at resuscitation decisions to look at the whole picture: this includes respect for patient autonomy;

awareness of doctors' decision rights; the success or futility rates; the cost implications of futile resuscitation; the time and other resources resuscitation uses; the underlying disease processes which the patient may be suffering from; and whether it is more realistic to aim to achieve a 'good death' with dignity and good symptom control. In this context, and with the majority of patients not understanding the full details and implications of true CPR, it is deemed futile, the doctor in charge of that patient's care should explain this to the patient along with the rationale behind it and then issue a DNAR order (Randall, 2003). Discussion about resuscitation status does not mean asking patients what they want: it can mean only explaining why or why not. Most patients will not understand how successful resuscitation will be in certain situations, and therefore it is important that they are not given an option to have it if this option is not feasible.

Medical paternalism is the term given to explain why doctors' decisions may take over a patient's treatment decisions. Orentlicher (1992) argues that often doctors may come to influence patient's own decisions, including end-of-life ones. Doctors may act on their own values because they are unaware of the patient's preferences, and this includes resuscitation. Perhaps this is because it makes the doctors feel uncomfortable to discuss it, or because they do not consider the patient's wishes to be important. Perhaps they feel it will cause the patient to give up all hope and thus compromise their recovery if they are told they may be in the terminal stages of their illness. Doctors also may not talk to patients because they can legally make the treatment decision themselves. Some patients and their family carers would prefer their doctors to decide for them, but their views still need to be considered. Doctors may also need to override the patient's preference for a futile treatment for their safety and for their beneficence. But often doctors make decisions because some treatments are not possible and the patient would probably not understand why: so they make the decision themselves based on their own risk – benefit calculation. When doctors do engage in end-of-life discussions with patients, they tend to do it with patients who are most like themselves, more intelligent and better educated (Waitzkin, 1984; Levy, 1985). However, for some end of life treatment decisions it may be possible for the patient themselves to have some involvement, with discussion including the percentages of success and failure, and effects on quality of life. Orentlicher (1992) argues that rather than letting patients decide everything without the benefit of professional knowledge, there must be informed consent and patient inclusion.

Case study 4

Mrs Brown is a 72-year-old woman with metastatic cancer and the primary is unknown; she was recently told her diagnosis. She was alone: her son was slightly delayed getting to the hospital and the doctor felt he did not have time to wait for him. Mrs Brown is a little deaf and so thinks she heard something about 'metastatic' but is not sure, also she does not know what this means. The doctor, straight away after telling her she has a 'growth which is a tumour' then asks her: 'If your heart stops, would you like us to resuscitate you?' Having been a great fan of any medical programmes on the TV, Mrs Brown recalls seeing several attempts at what she thought was resuscitation: chest compressions and a few shocks to the heart. She feels that this would be OK to experience and certainly wouldn't be too hard on her. Although she is in her 70s, she wants to live a little longer. As the doctor has offered her resuscitation, it must be appropriate for her. Also she only has a 'tumour' it doesn't seem to be anything serious. She says yes to this.

Her son turns up later on. Mrs Brown tells him she only has a tumour, and that they have said they will be happy to resuscitate her, so at least that's good news.

Over the next few days, Mrs Brown becomes unwell, and appears to dete-riorate very quickly. She develops a chest infection which does not respond well to intravenous antibiotics. Her son, although concerned, does not realise she has cancer. He assumes she has a benign lump, a tumour. And anyway, if her heart stops she can be resuscitated. Mrs Brown becomes extremely unwell and actually appears, to the nurses, to become terminal. Her breathing becomes very laboured one afternoon. The nurses looking after Mrs Brown assume her son is aware of how unwell she is, but because Mrs Brown has requested resuscitation they are aware if anything happens they need to start basic life support and call the crash team. One of the nurses asks the doctor whether he can make Mrs Brown a DNAR order but the doctor says he cannot do this as it is her own wish to be resusci-tated, and after all the patient has rights and he does not want to be sued by her son for neglect. Mrs Brown suddenly suffers a cardiac arrest. Basic life support is immediately started on the frail, dying Mrs Brown whilst her son is present. He is obviously distressed but feels that the resuscitation will be successful. He is taken into the day room and has to wait on his own whilst he sees lots of extra doctors and other important looking people run down the corridor into his mother's ward. He waits there, anxiously, for 10 minutes. Suddenly a doctor joins him: he says he is Mrs Brown's registrar. He explains that Mrs Brown was very unwell and unfortunately did not survive. Her heart and lungs were too weak from her cancer and also from the chest infection. The son is shocked: he assumed his mother would improve and says he was not aware she had cancer, that he was not told this and neither was his mother. He asks the doctor what they have done wrong: his mother was offered resuscitation and so why was it not success-ful? The doctor explains again that her heart was too weak. The son becomes very angry: he shouts at the doctor and states that she should not have been offered resuscitation if her body was too frail to be brought back to life. The doctor accepts his anger and apologises to the son: he feels he cannot let his junior colleague down but also realises a mistake has been made.

Two weeks later, after his mother's funeral, the son writes a long letter of complaint to the hospital. He has since realised his mother was dying and should not have been resuscitated. He feels his mother did not have a peaceful death.

This case study shows how offering the patient the choice of whether to be resuscitated or not was inappropriate, and it certainly was not in her best interests to maintain this decision when Mrs Brown became unwell. Her son went on to suffer severe emotional trauma and probable morbid grief reactions because he felt he had not protected his mother enough. The correct way to have dealt with this situation would have been either to decide that Mrs Brown was too frail for resuscitation to be successful, or if there was felt to be some chance of success to wait until her son turned up and then discuss it, using informed consent, to establish whether she wanted to be resuscitated. This would include explaining what resuscitation involves and what it does *not* involve. If Mrs Brown decided she wanted to be resuscitated because she felt she had a good quality of life to come back to initially, this would have been appropriate. However, as she become more unwell it should have been explained to her that her deterioration would mean that resuscitation would not be successful or acceptable. There would also need to be assurances given to her and her son of being referred to the hospital palliative care team to ensure as supportive and comfortable a death, in the most appropriate place, as possible. This whole approach would have prevented Mrs Brown's undignified death, her son's distress and following morbid grief, and would have meant the ward and medical staff would have provided Mrs Brown with a 'good death'.

A way of determining whether it is legitimate not to carry out a certain intervention is to examine it in terms of 'ordinary' and 'extraordinary' means (Singleton and McLaren, 1995). 'Ordinary means', when applied, tends to include means or interventions which are not seen as excessive or heroic, are more common and tend to be less expensive. 'Extraordinary means', when applied, means the opposite: highly medicalised, use of high-tech medical equipment, and uses of interventions which may seem to be preserving life at great lengths. In terms of resuscitation, in certain circumstances, it would be seen as extraordinary means when a patient is dying from a terminal event. However, it would not be seen as such for a person who suffered a sudden, unexpected cardiac arrest from which there was at least a small chance of success. However, these are subjective terms: what one person sees as ordinary may seem extraordinary to another.

Case study 5

Mrs Jones is admitted to hospital and her diagnosis is explained to her whilst her son is present with her. The doctor (a senior house officer; SHO) is the most senior member of his medical team at the time, and he feels that Mrs Jones, although she has metastatic cancer, is actually quite well for her age and disease status. He decides not to worry her with discussing resuscitation status as she seems quite stable at present, and he feels he would rather let the consultant discuss it with her when he returns from conference in two days' time. After the doctor has left them alone, Mrs Jones and her son discuss how glad they were that she decided to make a Living Will, and Mrs Jones says she will let the doctor know she has this when he next visits: she feels he seemed very busy and preoccupied when he left so she would rather not bother him with it at present. Mrs Jones' son says he will bring in the document from home when he next visits. Over the next 24 hours, Mrs Jones deteriorates a little but remains conscious, and by the night shift of the next day she is obviously very unwell with a chest infection. The SHO was too busy to visit and spend any time discussing resuscitation with Mrs Jones that day, so he sent the house officer. Mrs Jones was a little less well and had seemed to develop a chest infection; she was pyrexial and very chesty, also a little agitated by this. She was, however, just able to tell the house officer that she had a Living Will which her son was going to bring in; however, he had not been able to find it in the house as yet. Because it had not been brought in, the house officer was a little concerned about what to do. The nurses on the ward were asking the house officer to sort out a DNAR order since it was quite obvious Mrs Jones was deteriorating from the chest infection and may further deteriorate overnight. The house officer contacted the SHO and explained that Mrs Jones was not as well but did not mention the details of the pyrexia as the SHO was very hassled, due to being on-call. The house officer decided to discuss things with the other doctor later, as he had suggested, and told the nurse they would come back later. Meanwhile, the doctor starts Mrs Jones on intravenous antibiotics, slow subcutaneous fluids and regular PR paracetamol in order to keep her more comfortable. She also contacts the palliative care team for advice for prn medications for Mrs Jones, which is given over the telephone as it is now past 5 pm. She does not think about the DNAR status any further as she is very busy, is now on call in A&E and gets caught up in the busy department there. Both the house officer and the SHO take for granted that the nurses on the ward will remind them to make the DNAR status for Mrs Jones when it seems appropriate. However, there is an agency nurse looking after Mrs Jones that night; she is unfamiliar with hospital policies and procedures, and is not told that a DNAR status has not been made for Mrs Jones. The nurse assumes that it would be appropriate for Mrs Jones to be resuscitated as she is not dying yet, she simply has a bad chest infection, which is being treated anyway. The agency nurse feels it is appropriate for Mrs Jones to have the IV antibiotics and fluids as she is very settled and apyrexial, and seems a little brighter (she had had one dose of IV antibiotics and one dose of PR paracetamol). Mrs Jones' son visits later and agrees his mother is looking much better. He was not present when the doctor reviewed his mother today but his mother was able to tell him she had told her about the Living Will, so it would not be a problem. Mrs Jones deteriorates and despite the nurses asking the on-call doctors to make a DNAR order, this is refused as the doctor is very busy and does not feel senior enough, or that he knows Mrs Jones's case well enough. The nurses also request that the fluids be stopped as Mrs Jones is developing terminal secretions and after contacting the hospice this is what has been suggested. Again, the doctor is not keen to do this as he is still very busy and feels that as they have only just been started the nurses should continue them, Mrs Jones dies suddenly at 0600 the next day. Her son went home to get some rest at 0200, saying he would return in the morning, and asking the staff to ring him if there was any change. The only indication that Mrs Jones has deteriorated is her sudden death at 0600. The night staff, not finding a DNAR status, begin resuscitating Mrs Jones and call the crash team. They also ring her son and tell him that Mrs Jones has suddenly deteriorated and that the doctors are with her. He quickly gets dressed and comes to the hospital, arriving 10 minutes later. The nurse explains the doctors are still with his mother but that she is very unwell. Her son waits in the nurses' office on the ward, and is given a cup of tea by the healthcare assistant. He is not aware that the doctors are resuscitating his mother, assuming they are reviewing the antibiotics. Shortly after this, the lead of the crash team decides this is a terminal event and agrees they should stop resuscitating her. The nurse tells Mr Jones his mother has died. He does not realise she has had resuscitation attempted on her. The doctors come on duty the next morning and find that Mrs Jones has had resuscitation attempted on her. The house officer was surprised Mrs Jones had died so quickly but felt that it was appropriate to have resuscitated her as they had not asked Mrs Jones what she would like to do, and had not seen the Living Will. The nurses are upset that Mrs Jones was resuscitated since she had widespread cancer and was very frail with a chest infection. The ward manager follows things up from a nursing point of view. The crash team contact Mrs Jones's doctors and tell them in no uncertain terms that she was not appropriate to resuscitate and could they make sure next time that in similar cases a DNAR status is made. The doctors are confused as Mrs Jones was frail and unwell but had not seemed imminently terminal when they left the ward the previous day. They are angry with the nurses that no one had got the on-call doctor to make a DNAR status overnight, and the night staff are contacted at home and told to make a statement. The night staff are upset as they had not had warning of Mrs Jones deterioration until she had died suddenly and had felt it would be better for her medical team, rather than an on-call doctor, to make the resuscitation decision, so had not tried to discuss it with the ward on-call doctor. The SHO is angry with the house officer for starting antibiotics and fluids if Mrs Jones was dying. Mrs Jones' son does not realise what the circumstances behind his mother's death are. He is very confused and is not sure who he should speak to about it.

Note how the house officer and agency nurse, as well as the ward nurses, were not expecting Mrs Smith to suddenly deteriorate and die. No DNAR status had been made as no one realised she was likely to die suddenly. Notice how the antibiotics had been started and this was felt to be appropriate. Notice how the nurses did not feel that resuscitation was appropriate for Mrs Jones when she started to deteriorate, but that Mrs Jones' doctors had felt it was appropriate the evening before because she was quite well, although very frail. The terms 'ordinary' and 'extraordinary' are subjective, even when certain situations seem quite obvious. Despite the Living Will (which no one had seen), all the staff felt there was time to sort this decision out later on. The Living Will was not brought in and so could not be recognised; however, even in this situation, because Mrs Jones was frail, it may have alerted the doctors to realise she would not want 'extraordinary' means to keep her alive and may therefore not want resuscitation. It would have been a good time to have explained this to her in her frail state. The ward staff felt it was not appropriate to have resuscitated Mrs Smith when she suddenly died, neither would her son, if he had known, because he felt this would be extraordinary means. The house officer felt it would be appropriate to resuscitate Mrs Jones anyway, since no one had asked Mrs Jones what she wanted done in those circumstances and had not really taken on board the information about the Living Will since the patient did not have it with her. Notice how CPR seemed appropriate to the house officer, but the SHO would not have wanted this. No one thought that Mrs Smith may die suddenly despite the fact she was frail and then had developed a chest infection. The on-call doctor overnight considered the fluids were appropriate, whereas the ward nurses and the hospice did not. Notice how what one person sees as appropriate is not seen as such by another. This case study points out how vital it is to never leave important discussions because of being busy and never assume that everyone will feel the same way about what ordinary and what extraordinary means.

    In conclusion, Faber-Langandoen (1991) sums the issues presented in this chapter very adequately:

Physicians have an obligation to offer treatment consistent with the goals of medicine. A treatment that transiently prolongs life in the hospital, particularly the life of a patient dying of an irreversible disease, or relieving suffering: such a treatment is futile. Recommending that physicians not be required to offer resuscitation to the dying patient with metastatic cancer is not a return to the silent paternalism of medical practice before the 1960s. It is not fuelled by concerns over the rising costs or a nihilistic attitude that the patient with metastatic cancer would be better off dead. If we broaden the goals of medicine to include prolonging life as long as possible regardless of the patient's health, medicine incurs great costs. We violate the principle of truth telling if we present resuscitation as a way to regain health. We leave families with the perception that to consent to a DNR order is to stop short of doing everything, and patients with the sense fighting to the end is defined by attempts at resuscitation. We require our house staff to attend the dying cancer patient with defibrillators and endotracheal tubes. While communication and patient autonomy remain of fundamental importance, physicians must propose treatments that do not work, and CPR does not work in patients with metastatic cancer. To suggest otherwise to patients damages the integrity of medicine and does great harm to patients and to their physicians alike.

In summary, if there is any chance resuscitation may be successful, that is, the cardiorespiratory arrest is unexpected, it should be discussed with patients and their views should be sought. If cardiac arrest is expected as a terminal event then the patient should be told it is not appropriate, given the rationale why, and told what care will be given to them to ensure a good death, instead of resuscitation.

4 Cultural and religious influences, including the 'sick role', on healthcare and resuscitation decisions

The term 'sick role' (Parsons, 1950) was used to legitimise the lessening of any patient's autonomy whilst ill or in hospital, and allowed the doctor, 'the expert', to be the sanctioned decision-maker, with the patient trusting them, whatever. The sick role stated, in contrast to the biomedical model of illness, that patients were allowed – indeed, expected – to enter into this role as a temporary, medically sanctioned form of deviant behaviour and to succumb to medical paternalism. This meant the sick person was excused their usual duties and was meant to seek advice in making certain decisions. It was felt that such patients needed someone to speak up for them, in a situation where they may be unable to act as they would normally. It made illness into a culture, with its own set of beliefs and values.

Western society is nowadays much more pluralistic, with many different cultural influences. It is very easy for there to be a clash of beliefs and understandings which can underlie many problems. The same applies to hospital and healthcare in general. It is its own small world with its own culture, its own influences, beliefs, norms and values. The function of medical ethics is to make agreement possible in the healthcare system. Patients and healthcare workers are strangers who come from diverse backgrounds and possibly different subcultures. The patient is in unfamiliar territory, with often unfamiliar attitudes from the healthcare system. The patient may be contending with physical or psychological problems for which no cause has yet been found, which may then add to some already existing anxieties.

Today in Western society the sick role is now being challenged in several ways: by changes in how the public perceives doctors; by the recent increasing importance of human rights; and through the growth of equal rights. Patient autonomy is now very important in healthcare, and although individual patients may be unwell they should still have the opportunity to be involved with their own treatment decisions. When a person is ill for a long time, however, they often lack confidence about going home, and fear making any decisions alone. Therefore, it must be asked, if someone has taken on the sick role, even in a small capacity, can they truly make an informed, autonomous decision? Surely their decisions will be influenced, even a little, by this accepted, 'deviant' behaviour? Can they really be expected to enter into a true, autonomous decision about anything to do with their health if the hospital's own culture does not match their own?

Of course, the sick role is not the only culture patients will be exposed to. They will already have their own cultural influences from their upbringing and family history (Neuberger, 2004). What *is* meant by 'culture'? A common way of understanding culture is to see it consisting of three elements:

- *Values*: these comprise ideas about what in life seems important. They guide the rest of the culture.
- *Norms*: these consist of expectations of how people will behave in different situations. Each culture has different methods, called 'sanctions' of enforcing its norms. Sanctions vary with the importance of the norm; norms that a society enforces formally have the status of laws.
- *Artifacts*: artifacts – things, or material culture – derived from the culture's values and norms

> Culture is a set of guidelines (both explicit and implicit) which individuals inherit as members of a particular society, and which tells them how to view the world, how to experience it emotionally, and how to behave in it in relation to other people, to supernatural forces or gods, and to a natural environment. It also provides them with a way of transmitting these guidelines to the next generation – by the use of symbols, language, art and ritual. To some extent culture can be seen as the inherited 'lens', through which individuals perceive and understand the world they inhabit, and learn how to live within it. Growing up within any society is a form of enculturation, whereby the individual slowly acquires the cultural 'lens' of that society. (Helman, 1994)

From this definition culture brings people together who share similar beliefs, values and norms which they then pass on to others who join their culture either through birth or by other means. However, there may still exist some differences between individual members, and so Helman (1994) argues that there needs to be a distinction made between the rules which *should* be shared in that culture and those rules which actually *are* shared. Also, Simmonds (2001) states that the effects of education, geographic and social mobility on family life and cultural structures must be recognised since the second or third generations of a culture may be more or less willing, or able, to undertake the tasks of caring for the older generations, or of carrying out previously accepted cultural duties.

It may be seen from this how hospitals have their own culture, their own set of values, norms, sanctions and artifacts. Those patients who do not seem to share this culture of healthcare may be excluded from information-giving or even from respect. Healthcare professionals will usually only see a snapshot of patients whilst they are ill; this is a stressful moment of their lives and will not fully expose the true person. It therefore helps for the healthcare professionals to understand a little of patients' cultural heritage, particularly if it is different from their own. A healthcare professional's own way of caring for sick people in hospital will not be shared by everyone who enters that hospital or institution, and understanding how patients' own cultural values differ can ensure appropriate support and care. Healthcare professionals often see people in crisis, and it can be difficult to find out what cultural beliefs people have at such a time.

Nyatanga (1997) argues that a person's culture strongly influences their life, their view of the world and how to behave in it in relation to other people. Our values are learnt from parents, peers, society groups, schools and other institutions. Some people's lives are also influenced by religion as well as culture. Thus there will be differing values about treatment and resuscitation which will make each decision individual.

When working across cultures there is a danger that negative stereotypical images about people's family organisation and behaviour, derived from moments of stress and difficulty, will become the basis for 'everyday' knowledge about that person's community. Some differences can be quite surprising, such as family involvement: many cultures revere the elderly and will expect that they look after them in ill health. They will therefore not be particularly understanding of the Western use of nursing homes and may judge others as uncaring and unloving to their older relatives. Cultural beliefs will also influence how patients determine and understand their illness and how they deal with it: this will influence their own interpretation of any decisions made and this includes their interpretation of a DNAR order, of illness and even of death itself.

It is important that communication between those of differing cultures and backgrounds is cross-culturally sensitive (Iggulden, 2003). For example, Italians use many facial and body gestures during verbal communication, but the Japanese use very few. Also certain hand gestures or facial expressions can mean very different things in different cultures, and may even be offensive.

It has become apparent in recent years that many ethnic minority groups do not access hospice and specialist palliative care services as would be expected in line with their population numbers. The NCPC has raised awareness of this fact over the past few years, beginning with some work by Hill and Penso (1995) and through a seminar held in 2000. Several issues were raised as to why this might be. Cultural access depends on a number of things: communication, information about services, language that can be understood, and cultural liaison workers to raise awareness of the specialist palliative care services available. There are certain formal gatekeepers to accessing such services, usually GP's and hospital doctors, who tend to refer these patients to their local palliative care services. If this formal gatekeeper and referral service is not carried out those from ethnic minorities may feel, even if they learn about the services another way, that these are not appropriate for them or that they are not deserving of them. Not only should specialist palliative care services be culturally sensitive, but the aftercare provisions, such as bereavement support, should be as well (Firth, 2001). Even using the term 'black and ethnic minorities' can psychologically distance people by using skin colour, culture or religion as the reason why individuals may be seen as 'different'.

Traditionally, hospice services have been aimed at white, middle-class society and therefore many ethnic minorities will not feel part of their culture, and may not be keen to return or even venture to be referred. It is important for healthcare professionals and healthcare providers to be sensitive of possible cultural differences within specialist palliative care services in order to then be able to make other cultures feel welcome and deserving of them. Those patients who are able to continue living in their own homes may be able to access community-based palliative care services such as community-based palliative care specialists and 'hospice at home' services. These will enable patients to be comfortable in their own surroundings yet still have access to specialist support, for example, for symptom problems. However, specialists visiting their homes need to be aware of how different patients' views may be in terms of their judgements and beliefs, and be aware that their own body language may easily betray them. According to the NMC *Code of Professional Conduct* (NMC, 2004) all patients are entitled to good standards of nursing care, regardless of race, culture and ethnic origin. Therefore whatever the area of nursing or medicine someone is working in, there must be flexibility and advocacy, perhaps even negotiation, in order to ensure that any different cultural beliefs and values are understood and accepted.

Tied in with cultural beliefs are beliefs about death, health, and probably about cancer as well as other illnesses. These beliefs are based again on the influences a person has had in their life. Such beliefs and values will affect how an individual sees their health status and how they view ways to deal with it, so it is important for healthcare professionals to be aware of the fact that these attitudes will affect how they deal with the news of their cancer treatment where possible, of palliative illness and of death. It may be possible that some beliefs about illness and cancer may not encourage the person to seek the help of Western medicine, and this must be respected. However, the rationale behind the offer of such Western treatment could be explained if the patient is willing to discuss this.

Health beliefs are generally split into three groups according to Andrews and Boyle (1999).

- *The magico-religious health paradigm*: where life is based on supernatural influences and the fate of the world is caused by God, or other gods. Sometimes things happen regardless of what the person has done, other times that person may be punished or praised for certain actions. Illness is caused with or without justifications. (Perhaps the view of resuscitation in this paradigm would be to see it as inappropriate, because death would have been timely and would have been influenced by a more Powerful Being.)

- *The scientific or biomedical health paradigm*: life is controlled by a series of physical and biomedical processes that can be studied and manipulated by humans, either through mechanical or engineering means. Most people of the Western culture will belong in this health belief, and view medicalism itself as pertinent to this health paradigm. It includes believing that psychological health problems are influenced by biochemical means, for example depression is only caused by a chemical abnormality in the brain. (Perhaps the view on resuscitation in this group may be to accept it more readily as a 'cure' for death and to accept it as appropriate most of the time.)

- *The holistic health paradigm*: is similar to the medico-religious paradigm. The holistic paradigm sees human health as only one aspect of a wider picture of world health and harmony. Everything in the universe has a role and a balance, which, if disturbed, affects other aspects of life and the universe. Illness is viewed as an effect not only of a problem with the body but from a cause in the larger universe brought about by some sort of imbalance, for example tuberculosis is caused by the mycobacterium but in the holistic paradigm it would be viewed as being on the increase because of poverty, caused by increased malnutrition, overcrowding and the mycobacterium. Perhaps their view of resuscitation could be that it is either appropriate or inappropriate: *appropriate* because it may delay the effects of the wider universe which has influenced death and cardiac arrest; *inappropriate* because the wider effects of the universe on that cardiac arrest or death situation cannot be changed through resuscitation only.)

Thus not only are the views of a culture about death important, but also its views about life and health. How a person views life, illness, health and death will influence how they accept illness and death, and thus how they view resuscitation.

THE MEANING OF DEATH

How death is viewed by a culture can affect how people live their present lives and also by how they want to die. Bauman (1992) argues that in fifteenth-century England, people believed that what they did in their present life would affect their life after, something which is today shared by the Hindu religion. Because of this, he argues that people today focus only on this present life and place much intrinsic value on it. Also, many will want to focus on living as long as possible and in preserving the present life. This view is not shared by Davies (2002), who states instead that many people still worry about life after death and about the effects of their life on other people and society in general. Whatever the belief is, death will have some meaning to each individual, even if that meaning is literally that death is the end and there is nothing after it.

After death the body itself is treated in a socially acceptable way, according to local beliefs and culture, for example in Western society the body is removed from the place of death and stored until either it is safe to deal with it (such as in a case of sudden death or murder) or until the funeral directors are ready to help deal with it. Western society tends to opt for either burial or cremation, and usually the choice between the two rests on either the views of the person or of their family. Sometimes it is influenced by previous ancestral ways, as with large families who may own their own estate and mausoleum or graveyard. Often the body itself is seen as something unpleasant because it will begin to decay from the moment of death. Because Western culture is no longer the only view in Western lands, what happens to a body should form part of communication with either the patient or family before death occurs, so that their beliefs can be followed from point of death onwards.

How they view and value life and actual death may then affect how patients and their family carers view resuscitation. They may place great value on resuscitation as an event which they view as life-saving and possibly as even improving life. Others may have the opposing view and regard resuscitation as not allowing a dignified death: they may feel, whatever their age, that they have had a 'good innings' and that their life, however long or short, has been valuable but is soon to end. Resuscitation itself can also confuse the actual time of death, and some argue that it is a further medicalisation of death; indeed, requiring a doctor to legally certify death has been viewed by many as further medical influence over death itself (Page and Komaromy, 2000). How the moment of death is dealt with and what happens at the time can have great impact not only on the family but healthcare staff as well. It is not often accepted as a 'good death' by healthcare professionals when someone who has a terminal illness ends up being resuscitated, particularly when this is usually unsuccessful either immediately, or when the patient dies a few hours later. This view would most likely be shared by the family and the patient, and would not be seen as a 'good death' if they had been prepared for death itself as a terminal event. However, many patients and family carers will still ask that resuscitation be carried out, often because of ignorance or denial that death is near.

Roberts (2003) found that the age a person is when they die will give different interpretations and meanings to the death itself. The death of a child is upsetting because it does not fit into Western society's views of the natural order of life. This is true even when the child is an adult with parents still alive. Death of an adolescent, particularly through suicide, is deemed untimely and preventable, as is often death of a young adult. Death in old age is often viewed very differently, being seen as a natural event. However, some adults who may be seen as 'old' perhaps do not feel that way themselves, particularly if they have been relatively fit and healthy. And what constitutes 'old'? Is it from 70 years onwards, the 'three-score years and ten' quoted in the Bible? Some cultures revere their old, and may mourn the death of such a person more keenly. It must never be assumed that the family carers of an 'old' person will be less upset that those of a younger person. Although it often follows that the meaning of death of an older person to their family and friends is easier to justify, a younger adult may have been ill for a long time and their family and friends may feel, that although death was untimely, their long illness had been too much: it also gives the patient time to say what they want to say, to get their affairs in order, and to begin grieving. As a healthcare professional it is important never to underestimate how people will deal with death and grief, whether it is the patient who is grieving or a family carer. It is also important to remember even though a patient may feel ready, or not, to die, it will not follow that their family and friends feel the same.

CULTURAL CONFLICT IN ETHICAL DECISION-MAKING

With the multi-ethnicity of many countries there are cultural differences which may alter how ethical decision-making is carried out. For instance, Jehovah's witnesses do not agree with transfusions of blood or blood products, but there have been cases in the past where doctors have taken cases to the medical courts whereby parents who are Jehovah's witnesses have refused blood transfusions for their children. Also, Christian Scientists would rather use their own values and interventions when illness occurs than Western medicine or other more orthodox interventions. Just because certain people hold different views of health, illness and death does not mean that their views are wrong and it is important that differences are discussed and that the expected outcomes are not assumed. For instance, the Filipino culture does not agree with Advanced Directives (Living Wills) because they have a sense of fatalism, and planning for one's illness or death is seen as tempting fate. The Pakistani culture shares the Eastern philosophy of recognising the religious obligation of the patient to the physician. The ethos of machismo in the Mexican culture means that the views of the oldest male in the family will be consulted about consenting for medical treatment, even if they are living far away. A culturally competent model for such decision-making has been devised by Leininger (1991) and it identifies that when cultural beliefs and values are followed in healthcare then caring is meaningful and beneficial. Some readers may find it useful to examine these references themselves. If not, the most important thing to take away from this chapter is that healthcare professionals must be culturally sensitive, and self-aware when discussing care needs and treatment decisions with patients and family carers. Never assume how someone will respond to situations or questions. Always be prepared and open-minded.

RELIGIOUS INFLUENCES ON HEALTH, DEATH AND RESUSCITATION

Existing alongside cultural beliefs about life, health, illness and death is the influence of religion. Religion is complex in terms of form and function. Those who believe and follow a particular religion will focus highly on the faith they have and on any institutions included in that belief. It will enable them to make sense of most life experiences and will influence their way of life and their beliefs and actions. In terms of how religion affects a person, Faulkner and DeJong (1966) identified five dimensions of religion.

- *Experiential*: the religion expects the person to have some ultimate knowledge or religious emotion at some point and this is a subjective experience. The religion has certain expectations of that religious person.
- *Ritualistic*: certain religious practices are expected of that religious person and may include singing, prayer, participation in the sacraments and fasting.
- *Ideological*: this pertains to the set of beliefs the religious person must follow and believe in, in order to belong to that religion. This results in a sense of belonging and commitment for that person.
- *Intellectuals*: there are specific sets of beliefs or explanations or meaning to that religion. Members are expected to be informed about certain religious texts.
- *Consequential*: there are religiously defined standards of conduct which influence how that person reacts in a given situation, and influences their attitudes and behaviour. This aspect governs people's relationships with others.

These five elements of religion will influence how certain religions will view health, illness and death. Some religions may emphasise certain elements to the exclusion of others, and also may emphasise different values in terms of healthcare. This can affect how the healthcare professional needs to care for that person and their family carers spiritually and physically, and can also affect how the patient views resuscitation.

Religions have influenced how death is viewed by their followers, but the removal of death from the home into institutions such as hospitals, hospices and nursing homes does not always incorporate religiously sensitive death values. This has made death more of a complex process. If a person is unwell, or dies, in such an institution their religious beliefs will govern how they want to be cared for during and afterwards, how much intervention in the illness they see as appropriate, how their body is to be prepared when they die, and whether they wish to be buried or cremated. If there is no family to assist in any of these religious practices, it may be down to the nurses caring for that patient to be able to carry out what the patient would want. The following section deals with how the more popular religions may view health, illness, death and resuscitation. Of course, each religion may have varying views and interpretations on these beliefs and this section does not, by any means, attempt to cover all these aspects. It will simply try to explain how a patient's religion may differ from others and how it may influence interpretations of health, disease and death.

BUDDHIST

Buddhism indicates belief in Buddha. There are differing sects of Buddhism in the USA, Japan, Hawaii, Vietnam, Sri Lanka, Thailand, China and Tibet. Buddhists do not believe in healing through a faith or through faith itself. They believe in spiritual peace and liberation from anxiety by adherence to, and achievement of, awakening to Buddha's wisdom, and they see that this can be important factors in promoting health and recovery. Buddha taught that there should be no extremes of practice and followers should tread the Middle Path. In terms of health, medications should be used in accordance with the illness. Amputations and organ transplantations may allow an individual to live longer and therefore obtain Enlightenment, so these are acceptable practices. If there is chance of recovery this should be pursued in order to give the individual as much time as possible to obtain Enlightenment. If life cannot be prolonged to achieve this then death is acceptable. Calmness in death is meant to be the hallmark of a dying Buddhist. After death the body is seen only as a shell. Therefore resuscitation might be acceptable if it could be successful and therefore in a palliative patient who is a Buddhist, resuscitation would not be seen as appropriate because death would be viewed as inevitable in that individual's situation.

CATHOLICISM

Catholics believe in God and also that the taking of the Sacrament, when given by an ordained priest, is when the person actually partakes of Christ's body and blood. In times of illness they partake of the Sacrament of the Sick which includes communion and a blessing from the priest. In terms of medical interventions as long as the benefits outweigh the risks to the individual medications are permissible and morally acceptable. Catholics are mostly against mutalism of the body, believing in the Principle of Totality in which treatments are acceptable, if of benefit to the whole of the person; this includes amputations, biopsies and blood transfusions. Organ transplantation is allowed from live donors as long as the benefit to the recipient is equal to the harm done to the donor, and the donor can continue living without functional deprivation or of life itself. Members are allowed to take ordinary means to prolong their life, for example intravenous medications are allowed. But they are not obligated to take extraordinary means in terms of care or medical interventions. But what constitutes 'extraordinary'? As seen before this is a very subjective term and can be interpreted individually. It is also influenced by the patient's overall health status, the likely benefits and side effects, economic factors and the patient's and family carers' views. Euthanasia is not permitted and extraordinary means may be withheld to allow the patient to die of natural causes. Thus resuscitation in terminal illness may not be viewed as appropriate by Catholics.

CHRISTIAN SCIENTISTS

Members believe that God acts through universal, immutable, spiritual law and that genuine spiritual or Christian healing through prayers differs radically from the use of suggestion, willpower and all forms of psychotherapy, which are based on the human mind as a curative agent. Healing in illness is seen as proof of God's love and care. Christian scientists believe that God created the universe and human beings 'and made them perfect'; therefore human imperfection, including physical illness, reflects a misunderstanding of creation and is therefore subject to healing through prayer and spiritual regeneration. They do not usually use medications, and immunisations are only allowed if required by law. They are unlikely to agree to transplants, become donors or agree to biopsies. They are unlikely as well to seek medical practices to prolong life but as long as the person is alive they will pray for their recovery. Euthanasia is not accepted. Therefore resuscitation is a medicalised form of prolonging life and for this reason they may not agree with it, particularly in terminal illness.

CHURCH OF JESUS CHRIST AND THE LATTER DAY SAINTS (MORMONS)

This is a Christian religion which was established in the USA. They believe in God, but have strict rules for diet, which include no alcohol, tea or coffee, tobacco or recreational drugs. They believe God can use them to bring about healing. There is no restriction on their use of medications or vaccines, blood and blood components. If they lose a limb they could be fitted for a prosthesis. Individual consideration is given to amputations, organ donation and transplants. Wherever possible, medical science and faith healing are used to prevent death. But euthanasia is not acceptable to them. However, when death is inevitable their effort is concentrated on a peaceful and dignified death, and therefore they may not promote resuscitation in terminal illness.

HINDUISM

This faith is unusual because there is no common creed or doctrine shared by Hindus. There is complete freedom of belief but their overall distinguishing characteristic is the social caste system. Reincarnation is central in belief and the law of Karma determines life: rebirth is dependent on moral behaviour in the previous life, and life is seen as transient and a burden. Their goal is to be released from the cycle of birth, life and death, and reach what Buddhists call Nirvana (a state of extinction of passion). Roles and practices are carried out by Hindus within the framework of the caste system and focus on socio-religious ceremonies such as birth, marriage and death. Some Hindus believe in faith healing, others believe illness is God's way of punishing people for their sins. The use of blood components and medications is allowed. Loss of a limb is interpreted as caused by a sin in a former life. Organ transplantation is acceptable. There are no set beliefs on the prolonging if life. Life is seen as a perpetual cycle and death is simply one more step toward Nirvana. Euthanasia, however, is not acceptable. Therefore it appears that resuscitation in terminal illness may not be agreeable to Hindus as it would prevent their inevitable death, which is needed in order to eventually reach Nirvana.

ISLAM

Muslims, or Moslems, believe in one god (Allah) and that Muhammad is his prophet and founded the religion. They read the Qur'an which they regard as the uncreated and eternal word of Allah. Islam controls its followers' conduct through what is required, what is encouraged, what is permissible, what is discouraged and what is prohibited. There are no restrictions on medicines and even items normally not allowed, such as pork products, are allowed in the treatment of illnesses, for example pork insulin in diabetes mellitus. Blood and its components are not allowed but amputations and organ transplantation are for recipient and donor. However, the right to die is not recognized in Islam. Attempts to shorten or terminate life are not allowed, thus euthanasia is not acceptable to them. They see death as part of Allah's plan and that to struggle against it is wrong. Thus resuscitation for those who have a terminal illness may not be acceptable to them. Resuscitation may also not be acceptable to them, even in those who experience a sudden, unexpected cardiac arrest.

JEHOVAH'S WITNESSES

Their name means, literally, what is says: they follow the word of Jehovah, that is, God, according to the King James Version of the Bible. Medications are acceptable if required, but blood and any of its components are not: this is based on scriptural references. The right to die or to prolong life is up to the individual to decide. Euthanasia is not acceptable. There is no law against amputation and if organ transplantation will cause violation of the principle of bodily mutation they are not allowed. It is difficult to know what the individual's views on resuscitation are; however, death in the Bible is seen as normal when it is due to illness or old age, and thus resuscitation in terminal illness may not be acceptable to them.

JUDAISM

This is an Old Testament religion which believes only in God as the Supreme Being. A persons life is based on the ancient Jewish Law, which is an interpretation of the Laws of God as contained in the Torah and explained in the Talmud tradition. In illness, medical care is expected according to Jewish Law. There are no restrictions on medications if they are for therapeutic reasons. They can receive transfusions of blood and its components but are not allowed to take blood orally, such as in certain sausages or raw meat. Organ transplantation and amputation will differ according to individuals. The use of palliative drugs to relieve any symptoms is allowed, even if the negative effect of the Doctrine of Double Effect (death) occurs. The relief of pain is seen as paramount. However, euthanasia is not acceptable. Jews believe that a person has a right to die with dignity, and if a physician sees that death is inevitable no new therapeutic measures that would extend life need to be started. Thus they may not see resuscitation as acceptable in terminal illness.

SEVENTH DAY ADVENTISTS

The Seventh Day Adventists accept the Bible as their only creed and their beliefs are based on its teachings. They believe in divine healing, and also in healing through medical interventions. They operate one of the world's largest religiously operated health systems and institutions, including a medical school, collectively called 'The Health Ministries'. Physical medicine, rehabilitation and good diet are recommended in illness. In death there are no definite restrictions but they have traditionally followed the medical ethics of prolonging life and for this reason may find a DNAR order difficult to understand. However, as the Bible teaches that death is acceptable in old age and illness they probably may not believe in resuscitation in terminal illness.

Although the above only touches on some of the main religions it shows that even in Western society different religious influences may conflict with orthodox medical interventions, as well as cultural influences. Healthcare culture therefore may not be acceptable to certain patients because of their own cultural and religious beliefs. It is important to be aware of this when discussing resuscitation with patients and their family carers, in order to understand some of their confusion and fear if a DNAR order is indicated.

5 The role of the nurse and the nurse–doctor–patient relationship in resuscitation decisions

Whatever the setting healthcare professionals are working in they will be involved in caring for vulnerable people. This vulnerability may arise from a number of factors, including physical and mental illness, physical disability, learning disability, extremes of age or change of physical routine whilst in hospital (Wheeler, 2000). Whatever the reason for the vulnerability, it can prevent patients from expressing what they really want.

Many healthcare professionals may feel that nurses have no real role in resuscitation decisions. But the actual resuscitation decision, although made finally by the doctor in charge of that patient's care, should include discussion with the patient or their carer if appropriate and other members of the multi-disciplinary team. The traditional nurse–doctor relationship would have made the main role of the nurse in such a decision as *prompter*, a role which was still seen to be important in one oncology unit (Bass, 2003). This is an important role, as the resuscitation decision is one which should be considered for all oncology and palliative patients. However, nurses have several other roles in treatment decisions as well, and not only because they may be the main people to form a relationship with patients which could be influential both to, and from, them. Nurses may, however, bring their own values and beliefs into this relationship, judging the patient and therefore only advocating for what they themselves view as important. This may not be a conscious thought process for the nurse but could end up being an advantage, or disadvantage, to both nurse and patient depending on their understanding of the relationship.

The role of the nurse, and indeed of other allied health professionals in resuscitation decisions cannot be underestimated. The nurse is often the first point of contact for a patient, and therefore may be able to raise awareness for the potential need to make end-of-life decisions (Jepson, 2003). Henderson (1966) defined nursing as follows:

> The unique role of the nurse is to assist the individual, whether sick or well, in the performance of those activities contributing to health or its recovery (or to a peaceful death) that he would perform unaided if he had the necessary strength,

will or knowledge. And to do this in such a way as to help him gain independence as rapidly as possible.

The nurse is therefore uniquely trained and able to assist the patient. Nursing is multi-dimensional, interactive, inter-disciplinary and complex. However, to view the nurse's role in resuscitation decisions as only being a decision prompter is to undermine the autonomy and importance of nurses and their input with patients and family carers on a day-to-day basis.

In order for a true resuscitation decision to be made, there should be involvement of the patient and their family carer and the relevant multi-disciplinary team members. Other allied health professionals may have a closer relationship with the patient than the nurse. It is not so much who forms this close relationship but about what is able to be gleaned from the privileged time and information-sharing this relationship offers. It may be possible to learn how patients view their own quality of life from this relationship and then use this knowledge as a basis for explaining the rationale behind a resuscitation decision.

The nurse–doctor–patient relationship, however, may easily sway a patient's decisions about their care, including the resuscitation decision. Patient choice in treatment is a controversial subject since any treatment decision depends on the skills of the clinician (Thomas, 1997). Over the years, being a patient has been redefined many times, with there being more emphasis nowadays on patients' rights and control (May, 1995). However, unrealistic workloads and deeply embedded traditions of routine and task orientation can also be the biggest threats to patient choice and individualised care (Woodward, 1998), with less time being given to proper discussion and rationalisation of decisions. Imparting any information about cancer to patients and their carers is very stressful (Thorne, 1988; Ramirez et al., 1994; Costello, 1995; Morton, 1996; Deeny and McGuigan, 1999). The event of breaking any news about diagnosis, including a resuscitation decision, can cause a major impact on the physical and psychological well-being of the patient and can also leave the healthcare professional feeling stressed and guilty. Thus the role of the nurse is crucial in fostering a culture whereby both patient and staff feel supported through potentially traumatic events (Deeny and McGuigan, 1999).

A cancer diagnosis can cause many reactions in patients and their family carers, including uncertainty, helplessness, loss of meaning, a sense of failure, stigma and isolation (Maguire, 1985). These reactions are similar to those suffered in any other life crisis. There may, however, also be reactions of denial, anger, blame, despair and depression (Morton, 1996). By establishing an open and honest relationship with the patient, however, the nurse can enable honest expression of emotion in order to help them cope, however the cancer progresses (Deeny and McGuigan, 1999). As long as time is given to build this relationship, and time taken to break bad news properly, then however the cancer or illness progresses the honest open expressions of their emotions can help them cope. Breaking bad news can often be badly handled because of lack of awareness, poor continuity of care and lack of communication-skills training. The nurse specialist may be better placed to build this relationship, to offer expert advice and knowledge, and may be more available during office hours.

The nurse–patient relationship has been identified as having three or four phases. Forchuk (1992) describes three phases but the more-quoted works of Beeber *et al.* (1990), Pearson *et al.* (1997) and Peplau (1952) describe a four-phase relationship, with stages of: *orientation* (to those with whom the relationship will be shared); *the relationship identification* (with those in it); *exploitation* (of the relationship in order to set the boundaries for that relationship), and finally *resolution* (when the relationship's boundaries are finally set). These stages can allow the nurse to recognise that resolution may take time, and will not happen overnight. The nurse's role is to support the patient through this time emotionally, with information, good relations and with good nursing care to ensure the safety and security of the patient, both physically and emotionally. Through the closeness of the relationship the nurse may act as advocate and friend where possible. Having the nurse they know best present during the discussion when the cancer diagnosis is given can be extremely helpful to the patient (Deeny and McGuigan, 1999). This could also be the same for when the resuscitation decision is discussed, particularly if the nurse–patient relationship is in the resolution phase.

Martin Buber (1937) wrote much about the nurse–patient relationship. To simplify his work, he described the nurse–patient relationship generally in terms of an 'I–It' and 'I–Thou' relationship. The 'I–It' relationship is not a close one. Certain constraints dominate this relationship, such as time, and there are many limitations and boundaries within it. There is little sacrifice of resources towards this relationship. In the 'I–Thou' relationship, however, there is a great human element, and the nurse and patient both give time and effort to the relationship: there is little medicalisation involved. It may be that the two relationships exist together between one nurse and one patient, but there is an understanding that when the 'I–Thou' is needed, it is available. Taylor (1993) adds that the use of counselling skills could enhance this 'I–Thou' relationship.

There is a lot of literature about the nurse–patient relationship and it mostly supports the major importance of openness when nurses are relating to their patients' needs (Taylor, 1993) and that the patient should be seen as an individual with individual needs, not as a diagnosis or a person simply occupying a bed. Nursing actually takes place in the context of the nurse–patient relationship (O'Kelly, 1998). However, this relationship can be influenced by unconscious mental processes such as transference (i.e. what the patient brings to the interaction based on past experience: this can be positive or negative) and countertransference (how the nurse unconsciously responds to the patient) (Freud, 1925; O'Kelly, 1998). Symptoms of countertransference can include over-involvement with the patient (Hartmann, 1995): this could then result in a breakdown of certain accepted boundaries within the nurse–patient relationship, such as withdrawal, for example by referring to a patient as 'The arm in bed six.' (Holden, 1990) and using a stereotyped, routine approach to the patient (Yuen, 1986). It is possible that countertransference could manifest itself in the nurse as physical symptoms, including symptoms such as sweating and clenching of the jaw (Bonniver, 1992). All these responses by the nurse may cause the patient to be labelled as 'non-compliant'. Anastasio (1995) found, in a study of TB and HIV patients, that those who refused to take their medication evoked strong feelings of anger and helplessness in the nurse and these strong feelings caused the nurse to label the patient as 'non-compliant'. Anastasio (1995) continues that these feelings may reduce the nurse's feelings of adequacy and thus may justify why the therapeutic relationship has failed. If, however, the relationship is to succeed the nurse must understand and realise this countertransference, and then overcome it. Once countertransference is overcome, there can be an improvement in the nurse–patient relationship and an improvement in patient care. In terms of resuscitation decisions, the nurse must overcome any countertransference in order to achieve better patient support and advocacy where possible.

Mackay (1993) argues that the nurse–doctor relationship has improved in recent years due to deterioration of the public esteem for doctors, and increasing female equality in society, but feels there still exists an unequal balance of power between nurses and doctors which may be attributed to the differences between their education and training. This then causes issues in the nurse–doctor relationship that relate to this difference in the education received by both professions: doctors receive five of years university-based education, and nurses receive three years of school- and ward-based training, which can give rise to a feeling of superiority in the doctors and inferiority in the nurses. However, more recently, nurses are now able to undertake a three-year diploma training or a four-year degree training, and with the rise of nurse autonomy the medical profession has had to adjust quite significantly to the changes this has brought about; this has caused an overall improvement in the nurse–doctor relationship in the past 30 years (Sweet and Norman, 1995). This difference might influence who patients end up respecting most, and in turn, may actually cause medical paternalism.

Sweet and Norman (1995) argue that medical paternalism still exists in the nurse–doctor relationship because the relationship historically reflects the traditional roles of marriage, where the doctor tended to be male and the nurse female. This can actually result in difficulties between male doctors and male nurses. Savage (1987) found that doctors often avoided working with male nurses since it did not reflect these traditional roles.

Hughes (1988) carried out an observational study on nurses' and doctors' interactions and found that it is mainly the nurses who do the history-taking and the physical care of patients, and the doctors who tend to be in charge of diagnosing. Yet in diagnostics it was still more often the experienced nurses whom the more junior medical staff relied on for guidance and support. There may also still exist differences in doctors' and nurses' opinions, particularly between what they view as futile and what they view as important (Breier-Mackie, 2001). This can cause some medical paternalism, where medical views may seem to take precedence because 'the doctor knows best'. However, with the modern age of medicine, the more important values and principles in healthcare are patient autonomy, beneficence, informed consent and a relationship of trust between the patient, doctors and nurses. Nurses and doctors must work to the same ends, namely what is in the best interests of the patient, and then work with that patient to establish what these best interests are. There is no longer any room for guess work in modern medicine, and communication will be the best way to establish these values and principles between all members of the multi-disciplinary team.

THE NURSE AS ADVOCATE IN CPR DECISIONS

As noted before, the nurse is important in building a relationship with the patient. They are also important as advocates. Advocacy became a significant issue in nursing in the 1980s, the nurse being identified as 'the fundamental advocate' (Stutor, 1993). This is one of the points of the *Code of Professional Conduct* (NMC, 2004). The nurse must act as an advocate for the patient's interests and well-being. The values and beliefs that underpin contemporary nursing, such as holism and humanism, have advanced further the nurse's understanding of the need for a more personal, individualistic approach to patients' healthcare requirements (Dean, 2001).

What, then is meant by advocacy? The word is derived from the Latin *advocatus*, which means one who is summoned to give evidence. Advocacy rests in our common humanity and has a lot to do with human needs and human rights (Tschudin, 1992). But Woodrow (1997) questions who is the summoner, what is the evidence and how far can feelings be integrated into a relationship? In the *Oxford English Dictionary* (2005), the word *advocate* is defined as:

- to recommend, to be in favour of
- a person who advocates a policy
- a person who pleads on behalf of another, as in a lawyer in court.

This final definition shows that the original use of the word was in the legal system. Although the term is used widely in medicine and healthcare, it can sometimes be unclear and open to misinterpretation. Florence Nightingale taught her nurses to obey doctors' instructions and this became the norm in nursing for many years. This caused its own problems and led to an ethical dilemma between the nurse who wanted to help her patient yet obey instructions given by a doctor (Woodrow, 1997). The term 'advocacy' was adopted into the nursing profession in 1973, by the International Council of Nurses, and it has been made clear since then that the nurse is an advocate for the patient, not for the institution or medical team. The Royal College of Nursing (1992) defines advocacy as 'a process of acting for, or on behalf of someone who is unable to do so themselves'. When applied to the healthcare setting, this means patient advocacy requires the patient to be informed of their rights and to have access to all the necessary information required for an informed choice (Clarke, 1982). Rumbold (1993) argues that if a nurse believes a treatment is being incorrectly or unnecessarily carried out on a patient then they have a duty to make a complaint. This should then end the ethical dilemma of what to do if the patient wants one thing and the doctor another. The concept of nurse advocacy can therefore be accepted ethically.

But what about the concept of the nurse as advocate, legally? The nurse is accountable for her practice as well (NMC, 2004). Dimond (1995) identified four areas of accountability:

- public
- patient
- employer
- profession.

Although nurse advocacy is compatible with these arenas, it is not recognised in law (Mallick and McHale, 1995), and although the NMC expects that nurses will fulfil public and patient accountability, attempts by nurses to do so have sometimes ended in conflict with medical colleagues or employers. This has sometimes resulted in a power struggle because nurses are also accountable to their employers as well as the patient (Dimond, 1995). Some nurses have even lost their jobs as a result of this power struggle (Woodrow, 1997). Therefore the role of the nurse as advocate is only to inform and support patients in their own decisions (Kohnke, 1982). The NMC does not want nurses to be doctors' hand-maidens, as Florence Nightingale did, but to have a duty to the patient. This may cause a possible power struggle between nursing and medical staff, where some doctors may feel threatened by a conflicting viewpoint. It is important that nurses are not advocates for too many patients at any one time, as this may cause a conflict of time and resources, particularly if all those patients require the nurse to be their advocate at the same time (Woodrow, 1997).

The problem with the concept of nurse advocacy is that it assumes all patients need an advocate, that all doctors give inadequate information and that all nurses are capable of being advocates and are also capable of enhancing patient empowerment (Allmark and Klarzynski, 1992). Willard (1996) argues that advocacy can also be confused with beneficence (doing good), which dilutes the significance of advocacy in healthcare and would leave nurses without the special role of patient advocate.

The nurse has two major responsibilities as nurse advocate, in terms of resuscitation decisions (Saunders and Valente, 1986).

- To explore the competent patient's wishes and to provide information necessary to make decisions regarding resuscitation.
- To facilitate communication between the patient and health professionals, to ensure that any decision regarding resuscitation is based upon the wishes of the patient. If communication with the patient is not possible, then the views of the relative should be sought.

If a patient is unable to speak for themselves, there are other ways of representing their views: Advance Directives; the nurse's subjectivity; what others believe the patient would have wanted; and beneficence (Gadow, 1989). If the nurse believes resuscitation is inappropriate or is aware the patient does not wish to have it, they should act as the patient's advocate and raise it with the medical staff as soon as possible in order to initiate further discussion and the making of an acceptable resuscitation decision.

Case study 6

Mr Brown is a 70-year-old gentleman who has just been told he has advanced cancer of the oesophagus. He had no inkling at all that what was wrong with him was cancer, despite the classic symptoms of weight loss and difficulty swallowing. He simply thought he had a throat infection or another simple problem which the doctors could solve easily. He is clearly devastated and despite the fact his daughter is with him, he is becoming increasingly upset. He has been told that the cancer is inoperable and due to already existing heart disease he is not fit enough for chemotherapy. The only options available are an oesophageal stent to help the dysphagia and for some localised radiotherapy, and he has now received both. The doctors have informed him that resuscitation may not be very successful due to the stage of his cancer but they have said as there may be a small chance of success it would be his decision. Mr Brown is left to think about this and becomes quite concerned that he has been asked to make the decision: he would rather be lead by the doctors. His main concern is for his daughter who is recently divorced and lives away from him. Mr Brown is widowed and has no other living relatives. He is concerned how she will cope on her own after his death. Although she says she has friends he knows that she does not have many as she is quite a private person. He opens up about his concerns one morning to the healthcare assistant who is helping to wash him. Mr Brown says that he is frightened of dying, frightened of having pain and frightened of how his daughter will cope without him. The healthcare assistant listens to what he has to say and does not offer false reassurances that everything will be alright. She asks Mr Brown if she can report what has been said to her to the trained nurse in order to allow a referral to the hospital Macmillan nurses. Mr Brown eventually agrees after being reassured that he is not a nuisance and that the nurses want to help him. One of the nurse specialists from the hospital palliative care team initially visits Mr Brown on his own the next day and spends a lot of time discussing his concerns and worries. They broach the subject of resuscitation with him, since it was written in the medical notes that Mr Brown had been left to decide for himself. The palliative care nurse explains why resuscitation may not be successful and discusses the alternatives with him: of being kept as comfortable as possible and controlling any symptoms which arise. Mr Brown feels this would be a better approach and agrees he should have a DNAR decision made. Although Mr Brown still has some of his original concerns, he feels it has been useful to 'get things off my chest'. The palliative care nurse discusses Mr Brown's thoughts and decision on resuscitation with one of the doctors involved in his care and a DNAR decision is documented and signed according to hospital policy. The nurse later visits when Mr Brown's daughter is present and Mr Brown gives the nurse permission to tell his daughter, on her own, about his concerns and his decision about resuscitation. His daughter is very emotional and agrees it will be hard when her father dies, but wants whatever can be done to make him as comfortable as possible. This opening allows the palliative care nurse to discuss the DNAR resuscitation decision, which has been made, and to explain why. She tells his daughter that Mr Brown already knows the aims of the treatment he has had. The nurse discusses the daughter's concerns about her father and herself. She offers support through the carers' support group which is held at the hospice and also discusses with his daughter whether placement at the hospice would be appropriate to offer Mr Brown. His daughter agrees and after this has been discussed with Mr Brown, with his daughter present, the nurse arranges with the hospice a mutually convenient time for his daughter to visit the hospice and meet the person who leads the support group there. The nurse prepares the person who will be showing her around about what her concerns are, after getting permission from Mr Brown's daughter. She returns following her visit the next afternoon and tells her father she feels he would benefit from admission there, in order to give both of them support. Mr Brown agrees to go on to the hospice waiting list and is transferred there four days later. In the meantime the palliative care nurse makes daily contact with Mr Brown and his daughter on the ward, in order to discuss their concerns and to assess and offer interventions for any symptoms Mr Brown is experiencing. During Mr Brown's admission to the hospice he had his daughter receive intense emotional support both from the nurses and the daughter from one of the hospice family support workers. During these times his daughter feels she is benefiting from this input more than from group support, as she feels very shy about speaking in front of new people. After her father's death, which is peaceful, she is followed up by the family support worker from her local hospice who gives longer term bereavement support for her.

This case study shows the importance of recognising and helping to deal with emotional and psychological concerns, and how advocacy can help with this, either in allowing the patient and family carers discuss their emotions, in discussing resuscitation decisions with patients or in informing relatives about the resuscitation decision which has been made and why. Notice how Mr Brown was concerned that he was a burden to everyone but that once his fears were discussed this open communication allowed more expert support from the hospital palliative care team. They were able to offer help not only from themselves but from the hospice environment, which allowed longer term follow-up to Mr Brown's daughter. At no time was anything simply discussed with his daughter on her own, particularly the DNAR decision, without either discussing with Mr Brown initially or by feedback to him. This ensured he felt important and that his opinions counted. However, at no point was his daughter left out, but it was clear to her that her father's views were important. The role of the untrained nurse here was important: she was able to spend time with Mr Brown during his wash, which probably meant Mr Brown did not feel talking about his concerns was a waste of the healthcare assistant's time. The healthcare assistant rightly requested Mr Brown's permission before telling the staff nurse who was then able to refer him to the specialist palliative care team in the hospital. It is important to remember that any healthcare professional can be the right person for the patient to discuss their views and concerns with. It really depends who is with the patient when they are ready to open up, and also what rapport the patient feels they have with that particular person. The healthcare assistant was able to act as Mr Brown's advocate by being able to discuss his concerns with the staff nurse (after Mr Brown's consent to this); the staff nurse then became Mr Brown's advocate in requesting input from the hospital palliative care team. It may not be the specialist palliative care nurse who Mr Brown wanted to open up to: he may have felt he would rather chat with the healthcare assistant whom he had observed whilst he had been in hospital and was impressed with how she treated him and the other patients. He may have felt awkward talking to someone he had never met before. On the other hand, he may have welcomed talking to someone who he felt would be able to help him more, and was not working on that ward only. Nurses in particular may be the one person a patient opens up to as they tend to have more frequent contact with them and may actually begin to build a relationship with one nurse in particular.

Nursing models have been created to try and explain and guide the role of the trained nurse. One model of nursing care is the Roper, Logan and Tierney

(1980) model, which examines certain activities required for living, as well as lifespan, dependence or independence; factors influencing these activities, and individuality in living. These activities of daily living are:

- maintaining a safe environment
- communicating
- breathing
- eating and drinking
- eliminating
- personal cleansing and dressing
- controlling body temperature
- mobilising
- working and playing
- expressing sexuality
- sleeping
- dying.

Dying refers to the actual process of dying, not to death itself, which is actually the end of life. People with a palliative illness have to live with the knowledge that their life is going to be shortened because of their disease, and this, as well as how this is dealt with by the nurses, would be included in the activity of dying.

Although Roper's nursing model includes dying as one of the activities of daily living, this is rarely assessed or discussed with patients, mainly because Western culture is not particularly accepting of death, and because there is a fear it will upset the patient or cause discomfort to them (Birtwhistle and Nielson, 1998). However Broekman (1998) did not discover this in his study; rather he found that patients would, on the whole, rather discuss such issues with healthcare professionals, even if they did become upset during these discussions.

Nurses have many roles within their line of duty. Nursing takes place in a number of health settings and is a universally recognised profession. Salvage (1993) states the following:

> The mission of nursing in society is to help individuals, families and groups to determine and achieve their physical, mental and social potential, and to do so within the challenging context of the environment in which they live and work. This requires nurses to develop and perform functions that promote and maintain health as well as prevent ill-health. Nursing also includes the planning and giving of care during illness and rehabilitation, and encompasses the physical, mental and social aspects of life as they affect health, illness disability and dying.

These qualities and roles should remain constant, regardless of the place or area of work. As Henderson (1966) stated:

> The unique function of the nurse is to assist the individual, sick or well, in the performance of those activities contributing to health or to its recovery (or to

peaceful death) that he would perform unaided if he had the necessary strength, will or knowledge, and to do this in such a way as to help him gain independent as rapidly as possible. The aspect of her work, this part of her function, she initiates and controls, of this she is master. In addition she helps the patient to carry out the total program whether it be for the improvement of health or the recovery from illness or support in death.

The actual roles of the nurse are many, and it would be impossible to list them all, especially as nurse's intuition, which is widely recognised as existing in the more experienced nurse, is not measurable. The main roles of the nurse, according to Holland (2003) include assessment, planning, implementation and evaluation of any aspects of care which the patient requires; support to family carers; prioritising of care; documentation and record keeping; encouraging self-care of the patient as much as they are able; education of patients, family carers and other (junior) nursing staff; developing nursing thinking and practice through research, audit and critical analysis, and collaborating with other members of the multi-disciplinary team in relevant aspects of patient care. On top of this, all trained nurses are expected, where able, to be involved with policy and procedure development and in the preparation of reports. An exhausting list! On a day-to-day basis this hardly touches all the other questions, reassurances, emergencies, meetings, social aspects of care, and meetings nurses need to deal with. However, it is important to remember Henderson's comments about the nurse being 'master'. Nurses are very much in control of their nursing environment especially when staffing levels are at a more acceptable level. Nurses can actually, subconsciously or consciously, control what care they give to what patients and in what order: they are able to prioritise.

Much research has been carried out in the past about what makes a patient popular or unpopular, and this is still evident today. Patients who comply with all treatment, never moan about the care they are given and accept whatever the doctors and nurse say, are seen as 'good' patients. Those patients who may complain or make more demands on nurses' time than the nurses feel they should, whose family carers' complain as well, and who may accuse the nurses of ignoring them are often labelled the opposite of this: these are the 'unpopular' patients, the ones nurses will often spend less time with, will chat to less and may be slower to answer their bell. Is it possible that such attitudes to these unpopular patients may actually be detrimental to any healthcare decisions made about them? Would it be possible that those patients may have less intervention, and perhaps be more likely to have a DNAR order made without discussion with them? It is a dreadful thought, to think that healthcare professionals may do this according to how they feel about patients. It is certainly food for thought, for any one who has worked in the healthcare arena: that those caring for individuals, who should be non-judgemental and objective in their prioritising of care, may be unconsciously or even consciously influenced into making different care decisions and outcomes for those patients who are not as well liked by the staff as others.

A study by Jepson (2003) found several themes for nursing roles and the involvement of nurses in resuscitation decisions.

- *Consultation*: nurses can be consulted for their opinion as to the patient's quality of life.
- *Helping*: nurses can assist in making the resuscitation decision as part of the multi-disciplinary team.
- *Leading*: nurses can lead the resuscitation discussion, and initiate it, as part of the multi-disciplinary team.
- *Patient advocate*: the patient may ask the nurse to seek consultation with the doctor, as to their end-of-life choices.
- *Supportive*: nurses can have a supportive role, once the resuscitation decision has been made, towards the patient and family carers.
- *Supporting*: in the case of children, supporting the parents' decision in respect of their resuscitation wishes for their child, and supporting the patient and family carers through, and after, the decision-making process.
- *Initiating*: nurses can take the lead on resuscitation discussions with relatives when no doctors are available.

Jepson (2003) also found certain themes relating to the involvement of patients and their family carers in the resuscitation decision.

- Patients are most often *not* involved in their own DNAR decisions.
- A balanced approach is required as to when to ask the patient's views: some patients are far too ill.
- Information leaflets explaining resuscitation in plain language should be available for patients and their families.
- Wishes of patients and their families should be sought at the earliest possible opportunity (in appropriate circumstances) wherever possible: this should be one of the priorities of care.
- Documentation relating to the dialogue which has taken place between medical staff and patients or their family carers should be made clearer.

Bass (2003) noted another role of the nurse in resuscitation decisions. This is the role of 'ethical protector'. This was revealed in a small-scale study where trained nurses felt it was their role to protect patients from inappropriate resuscitation. It was felt by the nurses in the study that they had an ethical role as advocator in order to prevent inappropriate resuscitation which could then end in the patient 'suffer[ing] a lingering cancer-related death' if CPR *were* successful. The nurses felt they should advocate protection of the patient from this undignified way of dying, when it is deemed inappropriate, and should therefore ensure a 'good death' with dignity. As stated before there may be a need for nurse advocacy if the patient is being influenced by the sick role and feeling undermined by medical paternalism, and they may feel unable to make any decision about their resuscitation status. Thus the nurse's role may well be of ensuring patient safety and of being their 'ethical protector'.

NURSES' ROLE IN SELF-CARE AND SELF-AWARENESS IN THE PALLIATIVE CARE SETTING

An important role of the nurse, particularly when involved in caring for patients in the cancer and palliative care setting on a regular basis, is that of self-care. This is the phrase given to how nurses care for themselves, keep themselves well enough to cope emotionally with their work and thus physically with nursing. Many nurses suffer from 'burn-out' (a state of physical, emotional and mental exhaustion caused by long-term involvement in emotionally demanding situations), particularly when nursing palliative patients over a long period of time, and if this issue is not addressed it can result in physical and psychological health degeneration, such as depression, weight loss and lethargy. 'Emotional burn-out' can occur when there is deep disillusionment about a job, and it occurs frequently in doctors and nurses, teachers and lawyers who are impassioned about their job but feel they cannot make the difference they had hoped because of the system they work under.

Each nurse's experience of caring for palliative patients will be different and can depend on their own personal experience of death and dying. It also depends on each nurse's own way of dealing with the stresses involved in their job, and also depends on that nurse's own personality type. Lugton (2002) states that being professional and able to support others in the palliative care setting does not mean nurses become hardened and do not feel sadness in certain situations. Those who have worked in such areas successfully will realise that certain patients and situations will seem to hit home more than others, and may easily cause feelings of great sadness, insecurity or inability to cope, perhaps because such situations are either too close to the nurse's personal experiences, or because the nurse has developed an acute sense of empathy to the situation.

It is important to recognise that stress is not always negative. Stress is important in order to provide a stimulating, challenging environment. Stress can mean different things. The word comes from the Latin and was first used in this country in the seventeenth century to mean 'hardship' or 'distress'. Gradually, the meaning has changed, and at one time was used in engineering in association with strain. There have been several definitions given over the years, one of which is from Gaye (1985): 'Stress is the perceptual phenomenon arising from comparison between the demand on an individual and his or her ability to cope'. When stress is examined biologically, the hormonal control was initially developed as a coping mechanism, a 'fight or flight' response, which enables the human body to deal with tremendous pressure in life and death situations. Indeed, there exist many near-death stories telling of how people found ways to survive and made critical choices in near-fatal situations. This is because of the production of adrenaline and noradrenaline by the body, which in turn causes several important physiological changes to the body in order to allow increased alertness and readiness for the body to cope with that situation. The heart rate increases, blood pressure increases, blood is diverted to the main organs and muscles of the body, the pupils constrict, appetite is suppressed and stomach and bladder emptying is speeded up (sometimes through vomiting or incontinence). Although it can be positive, stress over a long period of time, can cause a prolonged 'fight or flight' response, which in turn causes all the physiological changes to occur but for a longer time than they are meant to, or are required to. Appetite is suppressed causing weight loss, blood pressure is raised which gives increased risk of stroke and myocardial infarct, insomnia becomes the norm, and feelings of stress and insecurity are heightened. It is important to prevent this stress response occurring in all nurses, but particularly in those caring for palliative patients, so that they are able to cope well with the efforts of supporting those patients and their family carers who may need extra emotional and psychological support on a daily basis. Some ways of preventing this burn-out can involve the use of distancing strategies, and making sure they are aware of their own thoughts and beliefs about death and dying. Wakefield (2000) suggested some professional coping strategies, including debriefing sessions for staff, where they are encouraged to talk about certain difficult situations they may have been involved in, and to ask questions in order to understand why these events occurred because of a patient's disease. These professional coping mechanisms may help decrease the occurrence of self-blame in nurses who have been involved in such events.

A person's own experiences in life can influence their attitudes when working with dying patients. Sometimes nurses and family carers may not be aware of how previous situations can influence them. Experiencing the death of someone close gives added insight and sensitivity when working with the dying and bereaved. But it is important for all healthcare professionals to be aware of their feelings in terms of these past experiences and not suppress them. The temptation may be to say that they are managing to cope, where instead the professional is struggling with certain situations, which will then also affect their personal life and their standard of nursing care. These professionals need to be aware of these feelings, and then know how to deal with them in order to be able to cope effectively in the future.

Lugton (2002) suggests that there are certain needs for staff working in such areas.

- Being prepared for working in the palliative care setting, and having opportunities to gain the skills and confidence required for working within this specialised area.
- Having the time, space and privacy to communicate with dying patients and their family carers.
- Developing self-awareness and knowledge of their own feelings and attitudes.

• Developing the qualities needed for effective relationships with dying patients and their relatives.
• Developing realistic expectations of what can be achieved in this situation.
• Developing team work and receiving support from colleagues.

The support of hospital co-workers has been found to reduce work-related stress, which can also increase work performance (AbuAlrub and Fawzi, 2004). This is something palliative care staff groups need to focus on, giving time at work for formal support sessions, either through professional support or clinical supervision. Even organised leisure activities outside of work can allow staff groups to relate to each other in a more normal, healthy environment and can allow staff relationships to be more grounded in reality, instead of just work.

There are specific situations which may cause burn-out: excessive workload over a long period of time; being too accommodating and not turning down work; not using all the resources available, or delegating, and taking on projects which are not possible. This latter situation can occur in nursing when patients are very unwell but are still for active treatment and resuscitation, despite not responding to the active treatment given so far. Avoiding burn-out involves rest and sleep, having regular holidays and breaks from work, using relaxation techniques on a regular basis, taking regular exercise and a balanced diet, and seeking career guidance in case there is a better suited job. Self-care may include learning how to deal with stresses at work. An important way of coping is to place work in its appropriate place in the priorities of the nurse in their life as a whole, alongside their other roles of partner, parent, friend, leisure pursuer and so forth. With accountability and advocacy the role of nursing is obviously very important. However, when the nurse leaves the place of work, that role of being a nurse should be left behind, thus allowing the person's other life roles to take over instead.

This chapter has addressed the role of the nurse–doctor–patient relationship in resuscitation decisions. There are many influences on patient care, including the healthcare professional's own life experiences. However, it is important to remain non-judgemental and impartial when dealing with patients and when being an advocate. This may then enable the patient's true feelings and views to be represented and respected.

6 Making resuscitation decisions: involving patients and their family carers

This chapter will look at who should be involved in the discussion of the resuscitation decision, and who should be consulted first. This can cause problems for healthcare professionals if not addressed correctly.

THE PATIENT FIRST

Ideally, the patient is the first person approached about the resuscitation decision, not the carers. The Patient's Charter (DoH, 1991) states that 'Every citizen has a right to be given a clear explanation of any risk and any alternatives before they decide whether they will agree to the treatment'. A person's decision-making capacity is based on their ability to understand the information given and the implications of treatment choices, and also how they can communicate that choice. A person's decision-making capacity can be compromised temporarily and can fluctuate perhaps as frequently as from hour to hour, or be affected permanently. It can be affected by medications, psychological disturbances (i.e. depression), co-morbid conditions, advanced disease and how the information has been explained to them. Many healthcare professionals will make the mistake of talking to the family carers' first instead of the patient, probably because it may seem easier, in case it causes the patient any distress. However, Broekman (1998) found that 90% of patients prefer to talk about resuscitation, and that in 30–40% of resuscitation decisions there are inconsistencies between the patient's wishes and the medical staff's perceived understanding of their wishes. The resuscitation guidelines state that where no decision has been made every effort should be made to attempt to revive the patient. Therefore every effort *should* be made to discuss a resuscitation decision in order to prevent unnecessary indignity and inappropriate care through inappropriate resuscitation. The guidelines further state that each resuscitation decision is an individual one and no presumption, including blanket policies, can be applied.

   The resuscitation guidelines state that a senior member of the team should discuss the decision with the patient or family carers where able. Unfortunately, it is often a more junior member of staff who has to initiate this discussion, a doctor who may not have even met the patient, but is on-call and has been asked to make a DNAR decision for the patient who is now deteriorating and dying. This is another reason why all resuscitation decisions should not be left until the patient's health deteriorates to crisis point.

   The resuscitation guidelines (BMA *et al.*, 2001) state that an advance decision not to attempt resuscitation should only be made after, 'the appropriate consultation and consideration of all relevant aspects of the patient's condition'; these include:

- the likely outcome, including the chance of success, from resuscitation
- the patient's known or ascertainable wishes in terms of resuscitation and end-of-life decisions
- the patient's rights, including the right to life and the right not to receive degrading treatment.

These guidelines also outline who to discuss the resuscitation decision with. This should always be with patients first, when they are deemed competent and able. It is only then discussed with the patients' carers. However, if the patient is unable to discuss such a decision (perhaps they are unconscious, under age or deemed as cognitively incompetent), it may then be discussed with that patient's family carers in order to seek from them what the patient would want in terms of resuscitation and active treatment. The guidelines also state that the only person who can make the final resuscitation decision is the doctor in charge of that patient's care. This reinforces the need to make advanced decisions for DNAR, as often a patient's condition may change overnight or at the weekend, when the doctor in charge of that patient's care may not be on duty. The resuscitation decision should be made by taking into account the patient's wishes, where possible and where appropriate. This is where the resuscitation guidelines may cause some confusion: they state that the resuscitation should be discussed with the patient, but also that the doctor has the final decision. 'Discussion with the patient' should be *not* be interpreted as 'asking the patient'. However, the National Council for Palliative Care (NCPC) (2002) adds to this confusion in one of its documents by stating, 'There is no ethical obligation to discuss CPR with the majority of palliative care patients for whom such treatment, following assessment, is judged to be futile, as such discussion in futile situations may be redundant and potentially distressing'. Indeed, Bedell *et al.* (1984) state that, 'In cases which CPR [cardiopulmonary resuscitation] has been shown to be of no benefit, as in patients with metastatic cancer, it should not be considered an alternative, and should not be presented as such'. It certainly seems right that if CPR is deemed to be futile that the patient should *not* be asked whether they would want resuscitation. However, it seems only fair to communicate to them and their carers that CPR would not be attempted, so that everyone is aware that the patient is entering the incurable, palliative stages of their disease, and to prevent any family at home calling the ambulance because they feel this is the appropriate step when someone dies, or because the gasping last breaths of their relative cause them to think the patient needs oxygen or paramedic care. Surely, with the advancement of patient choice, informed consent and human rights, all patients have a right to understand all decisions made about their care, if they wish to hear it. Most nurses and doctors may feel more comfortable, because of ethical and honesty issues, at least explaining to the patient and their family carers why a DNAR order has been made, although many healthcare professionals may find it too difficult to raise this subject with patients and their families (Bass, 2003).

Goss (2001) argues against the NCPC statement by arguing that DNAR orders, at any age, without discussion, are unethical. Certainly the resuscitation decision and its outcome can be discussed, with the rationale, and should be explained to the patient and their family carers. In the present Western culture which is tending towards more complaints and litigation in healthcare, and also because of honesty and truth-telling, it is only fair that any treatment decisions made should be explained to the patient.

Although the doctor in charge of the patient's care should make the overall resuscitation decision, who else should be involved? The resuscitation guidelines state it should ideally be a multi-disciplinary team decision. A workshop organised by the NCPC in 2003 discussed this multi-disciplinary team involvement further and gave some practical and realistic suggestions as to how to take this forward in the work arena. The NCPC stated, in agreement with the resuscitation decisions, that the doctor in charge of the patient's care should make the ultimate resuscitation decision, but that this decision-making needed to be carried out in a way which was not suggestive of medical paternalism. This is where the ethical principle of 'beneficence' can legitimately take precedence over respect for patient autonomy. Previously, these two ethical principles have appeared to *collide* with each other instead of *collude*. This is because professionals have superior knowledge to determine the patient's best interests (Beauchamp and Childress, 2001) especially when the multi-disciplinary team decision on treatment may differ from that of the patient or family carers. Disagreement between the patient, their family carers and healthcare professionals can occur because:

• The patient and family carers, and the multi-disciplinary team have differing values and understanding of treatment goals, prognosis and disease stages. Futility must be discussed in terms of the goals of therapy, which may differ between patients and medics.
• The patient and staff differ over quality of life issues.
• Patients and staff do not share the same attitudes about the communication of treatment decisions and who is ultimately responsible for this.

- Certain multi-disciplinary team members may have professional over-involvement with the patient, or there may exist a rigid multi-disciplinary team hierarchy which makes it difficult for those seen as lower down in it to be able to share their own views.
- Time and resource pressures.

It was established in the NCPC workshop that many of these conflicts ultimately come down to the roots of teamworking, and this includes things such as:

- The philosophy of care shared between the multi-disciplinary team.
- Appropriate representation on the multi-disciplinary team, enabling a broad range of opinions. There should be an eclectic representation of all possible members.
- Trust and openness between all members of the multi-disciplinary team, there should be an open respect for all views shared in order to enable true open decision-making.
- Clarity over who has the final decision-making responsibility, that is the doctor in charge of that patient's care, but that all opinions from the multi-disciplinary team are to be respected.

The workshop discussed other strategies which were felt could be employed to help multi-disciplinary team decision-making, including:

- Ownership of its own resuscitation policy
- Relevant training to include expected outcomes of resuscitation, communication issues, beliefs and expectations, legal and ethical issues, documentation
- Pre-admission information available to patients and family carers about resuscitation
- A forum for multi-disciplinary team discussion on treatment decisions, including resuscitation decisions
- Exploration of the patient's own views and clarifications of the facts about success and futility of resuscitation, and other treatments
- Understanding of the needs and perspectives of different professional groups involved in the multi-disciplinary team, and respect for these views
- Focus on all the end-of-life issues, not just resuscitation itself
- Honesty over competencies of those involved
- Second opinions of patients and family carers who are not happy with the decisions made and even transference of care to another doctor for a second opinion if required.

Reid and Jeffery (2002, also BMA *et al.*, 2001) suggest that resuscitation should be discussed with patients and family carers as part of the whole treatment picture, and in terms of whether it will benefit the patient as part of the whole treatment programme, rather than being viewed as a lone decision.

The views of relevant multi-disciplinary team members, including those involved in the patient's primary and secondary care, should be considered.

Once a decision has been made it needs to be clearly and appropriately documented and communicated to everyone involved with that patient's care.

It may not be appropriate to discuss such a decision with every patient, especially patients who are unconscious (Jevon, 1999) and have no immediate family carers; however, discussion may prevent future complaints from the family carers when a treatment decision may have been written in the patient's nursing notes without being discussed and explained to them (Rumbelow, 2000).

Case study 7

Mrs Smith is a 43-year-old lady who is married and is the mother of two young children. She was diagnosed with breast cancer seven years previously, and had had a total mastectomy and axillary clearance. All the lymph nodes removed during this operation were clear of disease. She was treated with follow-up tamoxifen and radiotherapy. She did very well in terms of her disease for the five years afterwards and was then discharged from the breast cancer follow-up clinic when the cancer was still found to be in remission. She and all her family talked about how she had been cured. However, recently she has become very tired and short of breath, anaemic and has some lower back pain. She is admitted to the oncology ward in her local hospital. Chest and spinal X-rays show a pleural effusion and lesions in the sacral bones of her spine. The pleural effusion is tapped and a sample is sent for cytology. A further CT scan shows lymphangitis which is exacerbating her shortness of breath despite the pleural tap performed. A bone scan shows bone secondaries in her lower spine. The doctors do not know how to tell Mrs Smith as she has been very positive since her admission but has told one of the nurses she is terrified the cancer has come back: she has talked of suicide if she becomes terminal – she does not want to suffer. So instead of the doctors talking to her directly, they arrange to speak to her husband off the ward, alone. He is devastated, shocked but says that he realises his wife was becoming weaker. The doctors ask whether he wants them to tell his wife but Mr Smith decides he should do it himself. They explain that they plan to give her some chemotherapy if she agrees. They warn him what Mrs Smith has said about killing herself. Mr Smith takes time to explain to his wife that the cancer has 'come back' and is now in her lungs and spine. He explains that the doctors want to try some chemotherapy. Mrs Smith seems very positive and talks of cure because she is going to have some chemotherapy. Her husband does not correct her because he also feels the chemotherapy may be able to cure his wife, otherwise the doctors wouldn't have offered it, would they?

Over the next few months Mrs Smith deteriorates slowly, despite the chemotherapy. Each time she turns up for the chemotherapy she appears weaker. However, her blood counts remain alright for her to have the chemotherapy, and although the doctors try to discuss stopping her treatment she is keen to continue and refuses to discuss any other options. She however becomes increasingly depressed as she becomes weaker. She does not, however, seem to show any indications towards suicide. She begins to have more support from the community staff, both district nurses and her GP, during this time. She refuses to have community Macmillan nurse involvement, saying she is not dying and does not want to be depressed further. Eventually she becomes very unwell but does not want to go into the hospice. On admission to hospital she states that she knows she is unwell but wants to be as positive as she can and wants to continue to try and be cured. As she deteriorates the doctors decide to speak to her husband about her resuscitation status. They sensitively tell him that resuscitation will not be successful in Mrs Smith's weakened state. Her husband requests she is not told about this: the doctors say they would need to tell her if she asks but otherwise will try and respect his wishes. Mrs Smith senses the nurses are being a little less relaxed with her and finally asks her husband. He explains, reluctantly, about her not being for resuscitation. Mrs Smith becomes extremely upset and is angry with the doctors and her husband that they did not discuss this with her directly. She feels let down by her husband and feels she cannot trust the ward staff anymore. She becomes increasingly withdrawn over the short time she remains alive and only really communicates with her children for any length of time. She dies two weeks later, leaving a distraught, angry husband who feels he has let her and the children down by letting the doctors discuss things with him instead of his wife.

One of the problems with patient discussions is that many healthcare professional find it hard to use the actual words, *death* and *dying*. So many other phrases are used, such as 'passed away'. Workman (2003), in a letter to the NCPC, stated that very rarely are these words spoken and certainly not written down. He also stated that many healthcare professionals will shy away from having such a discussion with patients and their family carers. He concludes by saying that unless all healthcare professionals become more adept at using the proper words for death and dying, how can the public who they liaise with truly understand that this is what they are talking about?

As regards giving the patient information about CPR, the resuscitation guidelines (BMA *et al.*, 2001) state that information should be available to patients as part of the Trust's available information, such as on information stands within a hospital or a GP surgery. Such information should be seen as routine. Once the public begin to accept as routine information on resuscitation being readily available and discussed this will then remove the distress that could otherwise be caused. Familiarity allows security.

The principles behind the designing of patient information on resuscitation were discussed by Farsides (2003) at another NCPC workshop. This suggested that the following principles be included when discussing resuscitation with patients and family carers:

- What is the purpose of giving the information?
  - to help patients and their family carers understand what is happening to them, or what may happen to them, so that patients are able to make decisions which fit comfortably with their personal wishes
  - to protect against litigation
  - to make policies transparent.
- What do patients understand about their illness and about resuscitation itself?
- What do patients want to know and how much is sufficient?
- What do patients have a right to know and does this correspondingly mean professionals have a duty to inform them?
- What are the benefits to the patient and family carers of being given this information?
- What are the costs of being given the information?
- To whom should the information be given, those who:
  - need it?
  - want it?
  - understand it?
  - everybody?
- How should it be given – to the general targeted population or to specific individuals?
- By whom should it be given?
- When should it be given?

(Further advice about developing patient and family carer information can be obtained from the BMA and RCN websites (see 'References and bibliography' section at the end of this book).)

The patient may have already stated their decision ahead by making an Advance Directive, or Living Will. These are now legally recognised and cannot be overruled by a doctor without legal advice. They will become legal documents in 2007 when the Mental Capacity Act comes into effect.

The resuscitation guidelines go on to advise that if it is clear a patient does not want to discuss a resuscitation decision it should not be forced upon them, and if there is a small chance of success and the patient is adamant they wish to receive resuscitation then this is something to be considered by the doctor in charge of that patient's care. However, if such a decision is truthfully discussed and honest information is given most patients would probably prefer a comfortable death with good symptom control, rather than a high-tech mostly unsuccessful resuscitation attempt.

Case study 8

Mrs Smith has just been told her diagnosis of metastatic breast cancer, which she said she wanted to know. She is, however, very shocked. The doctors ask her if she would like to know more details about the diagnosis and prognosis but she does not feel she can deal with any other new information today. The doctor requests that he speak to her son alone and says there are certain things about her treatment he would like to clarify. Mrs Smith clearly states that she does not want to know anything further. She would rather live each day at a time and die when the time comes. The doctor takes her son into the ward office and sensitively explains that his mother is deteriorating rapidly; indeed, she has deteriorated since her hospital admission a week previous and is now bed-bound. He states that her case was discussed at the breast multi-disciplinary team meeting yesterday and the oncologist present felt that Mrs Smith was too frail for any interventions such as chemotherapy or radiotherapy. Mrs Smith's son agrees that his mother has deteriorated rapidly. The doctor then gently explains the goals of Mrs Smith's care now, which are to make sure she is kept as comfortable as possible, and is where she would like to be. Her son states he would quite like his mother to go to the local hospice if this is at all possible. The doctor then explains that as Mrs Smith is deteriorating rapidly, she will become weaker quickly and will gradually sleep more and be awake less often, until she slips away in her sleep and dies. He explains that at the point of her death it would not be appropriate to offer resuscitation. Mrs Smith's son is shocked that this has even needed to be discussed and is adamant he only wants comfort issues for his mother now. Her son then returns to his mother and after a short discussion she agrees she would quite like to go to the hospice. The ward doctor states he will refer Mrs Smith to the hospital palliative care team in order to ensure a referral to the hospice when appropriate and to ensure support and advice for both of them through this difficult time.

Notice how the doctor had asked Mrs Smith how much information she wanted to know. He was trying to break the news to her at her own pace. This is important: if too much information is given too quickly, the patient will be unlikely to take on any of what has been said and more likely to misinterpret what is said, or forget it altogether. She may have refused to know anything, in which case he could still have asked if she was happy for her son to know.

He also did *not* offer resuscitation as he felt this would be completely inappropriate and futile. Notice how Mrs Smith's son was shocked that it had even been brought up.

What should be done about patients who are adamant they want resuscitation even when the clinical evidence suggests it would not be successful or appropriate? The resuscitation guidelines state that sensitive discussion should be carried out by senior, experienced, members of the multi-disciplinary team and discussion should be aimed at explaining the rationale behind the decisions. If a patient continues to want CPR, this should be respected but a doctor cannot give treatment which they feel is contrary to clinical judgement. Thus, another contraindication seems to have arisen in these guidelines. If the inappropriate action of resuscitation was *not* offered in the first place, this issue would not occur. It does seem much easier not to ask the patient in the first place, but instead to explain to them why the decision has been made not to resuscitate them in the event of respiratory or cardiac arrest because it will be a terminal event.

For adult patients who are not deemed competent to make such a decision, for instance those who are unconscious, or have severe learning difficulties, it may be necessary to speak to those closest to the patient, preferably their next of kin if they have one, to explore what may have been the patient's decision in this situation. However, in England there is no legal right for the family carers to vote by proxy for what they wish to happen to the patient if the patient is of age. This is only legal in Scotland. It should therefore be made clear to those being consulted that their role is not to take decisions on behalf of the patient but to help reflect the patient's wishes and views (Dimond, 2004). They cannot insist on treatment or non-treatment. If CPR is inappropriate in such situations the decision should be communicated to the carers so that they are in the picture. This is simply good practice.

Case study 9

Mrs Smith is an 80-year-old lady who has been living in a private nursing home for five years. She has one son who lives away and rarely visits his mother. His mother was left a large house and money when her husband died three years prior to her admission to the nursing home. She sold the house and invested the money in order to pay for the nursing home and has a considerable amount of money saved, in her name. She is admitted to hospital with shortness of breath and is found to have lung cancer. Her son is told and he requests that his mother should not have any treatment, not even a referral to the oncologist, since she is very elderly. He says his mother has always been adamant that she would not want any treatment for cancer if she had it. The doctors say that they will be discussing his mother's case at the lung cancer multi-disciplinary team meeting but that his mother's cancer cannot be cured. The son says he, rather than the doctors, would rather tell his mother what is wrong with her. He does not tell her of her diagnosis, and instead says she simply has a little bronchitis and should stay in hospital until she is better. He is hoping to get as much money as possible from his mother's investments and is worried that if he tells her she is ill she will sort out her will and give some or all of the money away (they have not ever got on well together, but Mrs Smith does not tell the nurses in case they think she is a bad mother). The ward staff and doctors assume she has been told her diagnosis, and are surprised when at the lung multi-disciplinary meeting the oncologist says he would like to speak to her to see if she is well enough and would agree to some radio-therapy. When he arrives on the ward and speaks to Mrs Smith she is shocked about her diagnosis, stating she thought she only had bronchitis. The oncologist spends a lot of time going through things with her and Mrs Smith is very keen to pursue the radiotherapy route. She thinks the doctors have lied to her son and the oncologist thinks the doctors have perhaps not told Mrs Smith in a straightforward manner. Eventually, when Mrs Smith makes a formal complaint it transpires what has happened, and the doctors have to explain to Mrs Smith that her son insisted he wanted to tell her the diagnosis.

If the doctors had spoken to Mrs Smith directly this would never have occurred. Her son had no right to even be told what was wrong with his mother before she was told herself. It is wrong for healthcare professionals to think that everyone has good family relations. In this case study it was quite detrimental to Mrs Smith and caused excessive shock and distress to her.

When a resuscitation decision has been made it should be documented according to local policy and any discussions about the decision should also be documented.

Costello (2004) felt that nurses used their intuition when it came to judging whether ill patients were suitable for resuscitation or not. He found that the basis of whether the nurses felt a patient was suitable for resuscitation or not seemed to rest on how ill the patient was, and whether it was felt it was kinder to 'let them go'. Costello (2004) found, however, that doctors were more likely to base their decision on the physical condition of the patient. Costello (2004) felt that nurses, due to having a closer relationship with the patient, often were instinctively correct as to whether resuscitation would be appropriate or not. Having this knowledge of the patient could be seen as an important part of the social management of death.

IS IT EVER ACCPETABLE TO DECEIVE A PATIENT?

Ballinger (1997) argues that using deception in healthcare decisions, either through deliberate means or through clever avoidance of issues, is a high-risk strategy. Truth-telling and honesty are basic moral principles, not only for healthcare professionals. Deciding either to withhold vital information from the patient, or by non-disclosure of truth, can affect the relationship between the patient, nurse or doctor. Such deception, if the patient finds out, could end in the patient requesting care from a different consultant, GP or hospital ward. If the doctor decides to discuss things with the family carers first rather then the patient, it could end in mistrust between the patient and their family carers, or between the patient and the doctor, where previously there had been trust. At this stage in a person's life, the patient losing their trust and support in their family, or vice versa, can have profound effects on the memories of the surviving family. Arguments which may be used to support the non-disclosure of information include protecting the patient; however, preventing the patient from 'getting their house in order' before they die, and perhaps causing them distress by their not understanding why they are becoming progressively weaker, can be the antithesis of a good death and can prevent the patient's needs being met. For nurses, the NMC *Code of Professional Conduct* (2004) states that the nurse must recognise and respect the role of patient and clients as partners in their care and the contribution they can make to it, and they must recognise that they are personally accountable as nurses for ensuring that they promote and protect the interests and dignity of the patients, and recognise that patients are entitled to information about their condition.

COMMUNICATION IN RESUSCITATION DECISIONS

How should such discussion for resuscitation decisions be approached? Any discussion involving end-of-life decisions can be difficult to broach and Reid and Jeffrey (2002) believe any resuscitation decision should be discussed as part of other treatment decisions, so that it is not seen as a separate entity. Although death is an everyday occurrence, in hospital and in the community, many healthcare professionals still often find it very difficult to know how to discuss it with patients and their family carers: what to say, or how to say it (Cooley, 2000). Good communication is based on the etiquette of showing respect for another person, listening to them and valuing what they say. Communication itself is a two-way process of trust and honesty between the patient and the healthcare professional. Talking about CPR decisions can be difficult, as many doctors may lack the necessary communication skills and may feel a sense of failure, of fear of litigation, or of distressing the patient. Maybe they fear a patient will refuse a DNAR order, and are not sure what they should do in that situation. As seen, the success rate of resuscitation in patients with advanced cancer is very small and for this reason, because the resuscitation guidelines state that a doctor is not compelled to offer a treatment they feel is futile, it should not be offered as a possibility. Remember, patients cannot demand a treatment that the doctors feel is futile and has no benefit (Thorns, 2000).

Such end-of-life discussions should not just occur haphazardly: there needs to be some careful preparation beforehand. There are some basic steps which can be utilised when approaching such conversations.

- The person(s) to carry it out: consider who has a good relationship with the patient, who they trust and who knows the patient's situation and medical history.
- Carry out a little research through the patient's medical records to see if they have expressed any wishes in the past, made a Living Will or shown any strong religious or other views.
- Make sure the facts of the patient's illness and situation are well known and understood.
- The person planning to lead the discussion needs to carry out some self-assessment: do they have any personal biases about end-of-life issues? If so these could subconsciously influence the patient and therefore that professional may not be the best person to carry out the discussion.
- Be aware of background facts in end-of life issues, such as ethical and legal issues.
- Practise good communication skills throughout the discussion, such as active listening and empathy. It is not a good idea for an inexperienced member of staff to practise end-of-life discussions with patients and family carers, but it may be worth them sitting in on the meeting to observe and learn.
- Clarify any terminology used: do not assume the patient and family carers understand what resuscitation means or even involves.
- Allow time and privacy for the conversation. Try to offload bleeps and pagers.
- Be honest with the patient.

Good communication in any decision-making is of paramount importance. Fallowfield (1995) found that cancer patients who received good psychological support experienced a greater sense of well-being and survived for longer. Caring for a patient who has been given a life-limiting diagnosis, or indeed has received any bad news, requires sensitivity (Cooley, 2000). It is important, at this point, to remember that bad news is any news which will drastically alter the individual's future, and the extent of bad news depends on what the individual's own expectations and plans for the future were, compared to what they are after they have received the bad news. In any decision-making it is important that all the parts of that situation which are pertinent are considered. It is difficult for anyone to make a decision if they do not know everything they need to know. For resuscitation decisions, if the patient's views are to be sought (i.e. there is a chance of success, their illness is not in the terminal phase) and considered, then the patient must, of course, understand the whole situation pertaining to that decision. This includes things such as what resuscitation actually involves, the likely success rate for that particular person and the possible complications and outcomes.

For those patients who are palliative, who are in the terminal phase of their disease, or who have a very poor quality of life, their views do not need to be sought. It has been stated by the NCPC that there is no ethical obligation to discuss a CPR decision with anyone for whom it is felt there will not be a chance of success. There are many professionals who would not entirely agree with this, because they feel the principles of truth-telling and honesty should be applied: therefore with a patient who is palliative, who is either in the terminal phase of their illness or very unwell due to other co-morbid factors, the best way to communicate the resuscitation decision is to tell them why a DNAR order has been made and then explain the rationale behind it. In order to do this, good communication skills are necessary, and the best way to approach this is with the same approach taken in breaking bad news. The reason for this is because for many patients the news that they will not be resuscitated will come as a huge shock, and may remain as such even when the rationale has been explained. However, for others there may be huge relief that this decision has been made. Because it may be very tricky to know how each patient, or family carer, will react it is best to approach the situation expecting them to think the decision for DNAR will be bad news, and thus to adopt the appropriate approach in discussing this.

A perceived lack of communication is a cause of dissatisfaction for patients their family carers and for healthcare professionals (Wilkins *et al.*, 1999) since the importance that has been placed on good communication skills comes from the fact that ill-informed patients are a source of stress and anxiety for healthcare professionals (May, 1995).

Von Gunton *et al.* (2000) give seven steps in ensuring competency in end-of-life decision-making.

- Prepare for the discussion: make sure all the facts are known, find an appropriate environment, make sure there is time to have the discussion.
- Establish what the patient and family carers' know: begin with open-ended questions about the situation.
- Determine how to handle the information given: do they want all the information or only bits of it? Patients do have the right to decline information and it should not be assumed that there are certain ethnic, cultural or religious norms. This step may need to be carried out before any other discussions take place.
- Deliver the information, sensitively, without the use of jargon. Kaye (1996) says it is best to give a warning shot, something such as, 'I'm afraid there is bad news about your results,' or 'I'm afraid we found a lump'. It is best to

start as gently as possible and then move in to using proper words, not euphemisms.

- Respond to emotions. Give time for this, as it differs in length of time and strength of feelings.
- Establish goals of treatment and care: this maybe less relevant in certain situations.
- Establish a plan with the patient and carers and explain what the next step is. This may be either review by a specialist, or referral to a palliative care team.

Peter Kaye's pocket handbook, called *Breaking Bad News* (Kaye, 1996), gives similar advice in 10 steps, which can also be applied in telling patients that they are not for resuscitation. (This part of the book is written assuming that the doctor will take the lead in this situation, as they are the ones to make the final resuscitation decision.) However, as stated before, it would be possible for any multi-disciplinary team member to undertake this meeting (and perhaps have a doctor present if possible; if not, the discussion can be reiterated to the doctor as soon as possible in order for the final decision to be made. However, many senior doctors do not always possess good communication skills, and should acknowledge this if it is so).

1. *Preparation*: Know all the facts about that patient's situation. Be aware that this may be a very difficult meeting so have the entire facts ready as to why they are not suitable to be resuscitated. Also make sure the patient has someone with them, if they want. It is important to set aside time for this meeting so that the patient feels they can ask questions. Give bleeps to someone else. Most important of all is to find somewhere private, if the patient is able to be moved. If not, be aware that ward curtains are not soundproof. It is good idea for the doctor to have a colleague with them, either a nurse the patient knows well, or another doctor who the patient is familiar with, especially if the senior doctor conducting this meeting is not well known to the patient and their family carers. Make sure, as well, that the person breaking news is sitting down; otherwise it can make the patient feel very intimidated and rushed. It may be necessary to set some time boundaries in order to be realistic, but if that is the case Kaye (1996) states that another follow up meeting should be made to discuss anything further, if the patient or family carers wish for this.
2. *Work out what is known*: a statement such as, 'It would help me to know what you understand about your illness,' is a good way to open the meeting. In this way, it is possible to establish what the patient or family carers understand about the disease, and how they see their present health situation at the moment. Other questions may need to be asked to make sure the full situation, as the patient sees it, is told by them. It may be possible at this stage that the patient and family carers realise how unwell they are, and request that they be well looked after and kept comfortable. This would show that they understand how unwell they are. Unfortunately,

the majority of patient discussions will not come into this category. More likely it may be that the patient either has not been told how unwell they are or has misinterpreted any information they have been told and are still thinking that they have a curable, or controllable, disease with a fairly good prognosis. It is important for the doctor not to take for granted that even if they themselves were the one to tell the patient how unwell they are in the recent past that the patient has taken this on fully, and to think that the patient therefore has understood what this means to them and their future. Patients only tend to take in a very small percentage of everything they are told in any medical consultation such as an out-patient appointment. It may be possible, with the patient explaining what has happened to them and how they see their situation, that the healthcare professional may start to see the patient's illness from the patient's perspective. A useful question according to Kaye is, 'What has been the most difficult part of the whole thing for you?' From the patient's conversation it should be possible to grasp their level of understanding of their illness; the types of words and phrases they prefer to use (such as *cancer* or *growth* or *tumour*); their main concerns; their beliefs about things such as drugs, or their views of death, and their expectations of the future. Some patients will not be very forthcoming, perhaps because they find it very painful to talk about certain parts, or all, of their disease experience. It is important that they are given time and understanding, and not rushed.

3. *Is more information wanted?* 'Would you like me to tell you anything else about your illness?' This is where it is possible to test the waters to see what the patient wants to know. Many may be scared to hear the full situation. If the patient wants more information, then move to step five. If not, 'I'm afraid to ask', don't assume they *need* to know. By asking something like, 'Are you the sort of person that likes to know what is going on?' they may consent to not wanting to know, but allow the doctor to tell their family. The family may equally be as frightened of knowing the full situation and may refuse to be told as well. If so, make sure they realise they can come back in the future if they want to know the situation more fully.

4. *Allow denial*: denial is a way of coping with fear and should be allowed. Many healthcare professionals get very uncomfortable about patients who use denial: they fear the patient is not fully aware of their situation and that they should be. It is possible that patients using denial are very much aware of their situation but choose not to talk about it as a way of maintaining their own hope, or as a way of keeping hope for their family. Never give unrequested information as this can cause huge anxieties. There are usually only a few patients which permanently adopt denial as a coping mechanism, and some will only use it in front of certain healthcare professionals. They may choose to use it more in front of a doctor because they would rather be seen as able to cope, or more in front of a nurse because they feel the doctor fully understands their medical situation most

of all. Denial can be challenged by asking questions; this does not mean that the patient will not be allowed their denial, is it simply a way of checking whether the patient does, or does not, want to know what is going on. Questions to use include, 'What have you been thinking about your illness?' and, 'Have you thought that you may be very unwell?' Remember that denial can be due to fear and lack of confidence.

5. *The warning shot*: this allows the patient time to consider their own reactions, and whether they want any more information. A suitable one for a discussion about a resuscitation decision may be, 'It now appears that your disease is not as good as it was.' This will allow the patient to realise that their disease is progressing. It is important to give the patient time between each piece of information given, so that they can respond with any questions if they wish. From this it would be possible to explain *why* their disease is not as good as it was, and clarify that they are now in the terminal stages of their illness, or that their general health is not good: whatever is the rationale behind the reason for making them not for resuscitation. It will then be possible for the doctor to progress to stating that he wants to explain what the aims of the patient's care are now. From this, the conversation can be narrowed to talk about what will be done when the patient is in the very last stages of their illness: that the focus of care is allowing them to be where they want to be, stating that any symptoms will be dealt with in order to keep them as comfortable as possible; that support will include input from the palliative care team if the patient agrees. The patient then has time to understand the aim of the conversation before the actual topic of resuscitation is approached. Use statements such as 'When you are really unwell, and very close to death, it would not be appropriate for us to try and resuscitate you.' The rationale behind this can then be explained if the patient wishes: they may, however, take what has been said as acceptable.

6. *Explain (if requested)*: 'Do you want me to go over anything?', or, 'Do you have any questions?'. The aim here is to make sure that the patient, and family carers when included, have understood what has been said. Use kind words in order to soften the blow of anything they may not have understood and avoid medical jargon: it may give the doctor a sense of security but won't help the patient at this point.

7. *Elicit concerns*: 'What is worrying you the most?' may be a good phrase to use to see if there are any underlying fears which the patient may not have already explained. It would also allow the patient time to ask any questions relating to why they would not be resuscitated. Many patients may be distressed but may not be certain of why.

8. *Venting feelings*: This is often where the therapeutic part of the meeting takes place, and the aim is to help the patient try to name their feelings. The idea is that is the patient can name what is troubling them (e.g. they are frightened of dying, or they are angry that they will not be resuscitated), they can acknowledge it and deal with it, thus leading to a sense of

control. Encouraging the venting of feelings is a good way of conveying empathy to the patient, which is much more therapeutic than sympathy. The doctor may find this stage difficult, as the patient may be very tearful. It is, however, important to stay calm and not to offer false hope.

9. *Summary and plan*: This is a way of beginning to end the meeting by making a plan. This shows leadership and support to the patient in a time of crisis. The plan should reinforce the individuality of the patient and of their needs. The patient may feel very concerned about dying in pain, and the doctor could say that they would get the palliative care team to discuss how they could be supported, to try and ensure as much as possible that this does not occur. There may be other options such as input from a local hospice at home team, or hospice care: the patient may need time to think about the options available, and the doctor may need to be prepared to tell them if any of their options are unrealistic.

10. *Offer availability*: This is often the most important thing for the patient and their family carers: that the doctor is available to discuss any of their concerns, or their choices, in the future. It allows patients to feel supported, so that if they do not remember all the details of the conversation they can ask; it allows emotional adjustment, which takes time, and it allows the patient to introduce any other relatives to the doctor who may have concerns of their own.

Kaye (1996) continues that good communication maintains trust between healthcare professionals and the patient, can reduce uncertainty about the future, can prevent inappropriate hope through truth telling and honesty, and can allow appropriate adjustment. It also prevents a 'conspiracy of silence' which can make the patient feel paranoid and threatened.

Although Kaye's (1996) 10-step approach can seem quite simple, breaking any bad news, be it telling the patient there is no more treatment that can be offered, telling the patient they will not be able to go back to their own home and instead will need to go into a nursing home in order to be looked after in the future, or telling them they are not appropriate for resuscitation, can make healthcare professionals feel very uncomfortable and can make breaking such news very difficult. Kaye (1996) gives some reason why this may be:

• It can make the person feel incompetent in their communication skills because they are worried they may cause distress.
• They may fear being blamed because they are the bearer of such difficult news.
• They are concerned they may unleash a bad reaction from the patient or family carers by telling them this difficult news.
• They may feel they are failing the patient by not being able to cure them, or by not being able to offer some hope through resuscitation.
• They may feel they want to shield the patient from difficult news, and offer 'unrealistic optimism'. This is the worst thing to do as the patient may cling

to anything positive that is offered and then be even more disappointed, and more distrusting of the healthcare professional, in the future when it cannot really be offered.

- They may feel awkward about showing sympathy as a professional, in case they appear weak or not in control.
- They feel powerless to control the patient's emotional distress, because they may feel used to having the power to change things positively (this especially applies to doctors).
- They may feel embarrassed about how to behave if someone becomes upset.
- They may feel they do not have enough time to deal with any upset the meeting may have caused (although patient satisfaction depends less on time spent than the quality of the interaction).
- They are reminded of the human vulnerability to illness which reminds them of their own hidden agenda of mortality.

Kaye (1996) stresses that it is important to use clear terms, not jargon, in such meetings, for example 'cardiopulmonary resuscitation' or 'supportive and active treatment'. These can mean different things to different people, and are not part of the lay person's language; therefore clear language must be used, and where jargon is necessary it must be interpreted. It is important to stress the clarity of information given, that no jargon be used and patients' understanding of the situation be requested. Patients need to understand all the facts in order to make a decision, or to understand why a certain decision has been made.

To begin the resuscitation decision conversation, Lo (1991) suggests phrases such as, 'Would you like to discuss what you would want us to do in case you become too unwell to talk with us?' Or, 'One important issue is cardiopulmonary resuscitation, or CPR. Let me explain what CPR is . . .'. These openers are much clearer than asking a patient: 'In the event of your heart or lungs stopping, would you like us to start them up again?' This implies the heart and lungs can be restarted as easily as jump starting a car, or changing a fuse, which it is not: it is important not to allow this viewpoint to develop for the patient.

Resuscitation discussion or any treatment discussions can easily cause family collusion. In order to deal with this, Kay (1996) offers some support as to how to deal with the situation of the family carers refusing a DNAR order, or refusing withdrawal of treatment, because they do not want any discussion with the patient to upset them, or because they are very protective of their relative and want to know everything has been done but do not understand that there are often difficult side effects from futile treatments. It is right that, legally speaking, the patient has a right to know about treatment decisions; however, there is a more sensitive approach that can be taken in such situation and which may assist to reassure the relatives. This is a four-step approach, but all of them do not need to occur on the same day; it helps to address the question of: 'Does the patient *need* to know?' And 'Does the patient *want* to know?'.

1. *Family first, with the patient's permission*: After dealing with the patient's main concerns, it is a must to ask if they are happy that the relatives be spoken to alone, and told of what is going on. Most patients are happy that their family carers are not being left out. If the patient wants to have the conversation with the family present then it is probably because they want openness.

2. *Talk with the relatives*: The aim of this is to gain their trust by listening to their request of not telling the patient. It is important to check their understanding of the situation as well:
   - affirm: 'You know best'
   - check understanding: 'What is your understanding of what is going on with your relative?'
   - check reasons for not telling: 'Have you had anyone else in your family who has been ill/had cancer?' 'What happened with them?'
   - check the cost of not telling: 'Is it sometimes difficult for you?' 'What are your fears if your relative is told?'
   - seek permission to talk with the patient alone: the main fear is if the patient asks the doctor what is wrong; explain that the aim is only to find out what the patient wants to know.

3. *Talk with the patient alone*: Start checking for signs of denial by asking them, 'How do you think things are going at the moment?' Then ask: 'What does your family know about your illness?' which often leads on to a discussion of the communication difficulties from the patient's point of view. Sometimes the family are right and the patient is in total denial; the focus can then shift to any communication blocks about other issues other than the illness and present situation.

4. *Talk with the patient and family together*: This step can be brief but is essential in order to move on. The relatives then are at least aware of what the patient has been told because they were present. The principle aim is to act as a bridge and help both the patient and their family carers to understand each other's level of understanding, for example by saying to the patient, 'May I share with your family what we just discussed together?'

Kaye (1996) also states that it is important to remember that it is only very occasionally that family do not really want the patient to know: it often means they are worried the patient will be hurt and upset by the news, and they would rather this did not happen. If the family realise that once the patient knows the situation, they will not worry as much when they become weaker and nothing is really done about why this is so, and that they can 'get their house in order', they may not feel as protective.

Way *et al.* (2002) states that in a situation of family collusion and family conflict, using good communication skills and negotiation strategies (such as education) and consensus building are important in order to build up the patient's and family carers' trust.

Lugton (2002) states that another part of good communication skills involves the professional being able to assess the patient's coping styles, by assessing the patient's understanding of their disease and trying to see how the patient sees their future. Lugton outlines certain feelings which the patient may use.

- *Denial*: Some patients may use denial early on in their disease, which may be helpful in order to give them space to come to terms with their diagnosis. However, if this denial continues through into the palliative and then terminal stages of the disease the patient may not understand why they are becoming ill, and then possibly blame the doctors or nurses for not giving them appropriate treatment and care. Denial prevents the patient from being given appropriate information about their illness.
- *Anger* is shown in terms of short tempers and aggression. This often disguises underlying fears and anxieties. When it is directed against professionals this may cause the patient to become quite isolated. Anger can prevent the patient and family from using the remaining time positively. Allowing patients and family carers to talk about their experiences and difficulties may help diffuse this anger by talking about their feelings and difficult situations and allowing them to feel that the staff understand of their difficulties.
- *Bargaining* may be used when the illness becomes terminal, asking the medical staff for inappropriate treatments or bargaining with God for a cure or remission. They may try complementary and alternative therapies, or dietary changes. It is important not to take away this decision making because patients need to feel some control over an uncontrollable situation.
- *Depression*: It is untrue that all dying patients are depressed. However, it is a common occurrence in such patients. It is associated with losses and anticipated losses, such as loss of independence, physical attractiveness, role relationships and life itself. Mood disturbances may be caused by physical symptoms, such as pain. If depression is not appropriately diagnosed and treated it can affect the patient's quality of life.
- *Anxiety* about the future, of physical symptoms, of losing control and dignity at the end is very common in palliative patients. Family carers are often anxious about how they will cope physically, emotionally and financially. A helpful factor in relieving some of this is by having a professional involved whom the patient and family carers already respect, thus making it important for a palliative care specialist or unit to become involved early on in the diagnosis.
- *Obsessional behaviour*, such as noting down all the details of their treatment and of conversations they have had with professionals, may be prevalent and is often an attempt to regain control over the situation.

Lugton (2002) continues that it is important to support the patient's own identity in advanced illness and to allow support from friends, family carers and fellow patients. These actions can help the patient in coming to terms with their personal illness trajectory.

In any discussion of communication, non-verbal communication needs to be included. Non-verbal communication includes tone of voice, body language, facial expressions, eye contact, touch, silence and non-verbal humour. Of course, this works between all those who are communicating, and is never one-way. Non-verbal communication has been seen as carrying four times as much weight as verbal communication (Henley, 1973). However, it is important to remember that the actual words said are very important as well as *how* they are said. Stewart (1992) claims that words make up 10% of communication, tone makes up 40% and the final 50% is visual. Argyle (1992) states that, 'Non-verbal communication is a powerful indication of what we think and feel'. Health professionals need to be able to read patients' and family carers' non-verbal communication and also be aware that theirs will be seen and interpreted as well. It can be very hard to prevent the face showing any feelings, and patients will quickly pick up any displayed fear, anger, pity or sadness. Although it may be helpful in some situation for such feelings to be displayed by the healthcare professional it will not always be helpful. It is therefore important to be aware of posture, tone of voice, facial expressions, eye contact, touch and silence. The starting point for any good communication skills is good socialisation skills. People who are used to, and enjoy, meeting new people will find that developing good communisation skills is easier than those who are more self-contained and shy. To feel confident enough to be warm and supportive to relative strangers does not always come easily to some people. But when working with ill people any type of interaction, be it for a palliative patient or not, should be sensitive, warm, and the healthcare professional should show an interest in what is being said by that person in order to develop the feelings of truth and respect.

INFORMED CONSENT AND MEDICAL PATERNALISM

Patients seek medical advice because they do not understand the medical facts and they are often vulnerable and facing difficult life-changing decisions: this means doctors need to adopt 'responsible paternalism' and help make the decision on behalf of the patient once it is clear they trust that doctor (Raskin, 1994). Doctors are seen as the experts, they should understand the success rates of what they offer, possible benefits and known side effects (Brier-Mackie, 2001). For this reason many patients may be happy to ask the doctor's advice in this area, which would sit happily with doctors explaining why they would, or would not, think resuscitation is appropriate.

Also, Orentlicher (1992) argues that doctors' own values can influence end-of life discussions. The doctor may act on their own values because they are unaware of the patient's own values; perhaps they do not ask what the patient's own values because of their own discomfort with end-of-life issues and interestingly it seems that the patients they prefer to discuss such things with are those who are most like themselves.

The resuscitation guidelines (BMA *et al.*, 2001) state that there is no right to attempt resuscitation on competent adults who refuse treatment, even if such a decision results in death. For all other treatments, patients consent to *have* them but resuscitation is the only treatment where people are offered *not* to have it. The aim for any treatment decisions, including CPR, is for there to be general consensus amongst all involved. In cases where there may be severe family collusion against an inappropriate CPR decision, legal advice may even be required.

In summary, many issues involved in treatment decisions have been discussed. The most important thing to remember is that resuscitation decisions should be discussed with the patient first unless there are any contraindications to this. It is as important to remember that if resuscitation is deemed to be futile the patient has no right to demand it. Therefore it should not be offered. However, because of honesty and truth-telling it may be considered appropriate to explain the rationale behind this decision to the patient.

7 Hope in patients who are palliative and have had a DNAR order made

It has already been said that truth-telling is the centre of any treatment discussions, but certainly in resuscitation decision-making, particularly if a patient and family carers cannot initially understand the rationale behind the decision made. Herth (1990b) argues that truth-telling may conflict with clinicians' need to inspire hope. They may feel compelled to offer some future hope in the form of a treatment option. Tobias and Souhami (1993) state 'Most clinicians recognise that the anxious patient sitting opposite them requires above all reassurance and a clear exposition of what needs to be done to provide a cure'. However, Baverman (1991) condemns this attitude by stating, 'Many oncologists recommend chemotherapy for virtually any tumour with a hopefulness undiscouraged by invariable failure'.

There is an argument for not discussing resuscitation with terminally ill patients: this states that such discussion reduces any hope, especially when something which is futile may be offered as a possible treatment (Manisty and Waxman, 2003).

One aspect of palliative care which has not yet been discussed is hope. Hope is a major element for palliative patients who have to live every day uncertain as to the course of their illness and length of life (Lugton, 2002). Hope is a nebulous, elusive concept, which has been variously defined in the psychological, sociological, theological and healthcare literature (Chaplin and McIntyre, 2002) and has been described as being closely related to spiritual well-being in terms of providing a sense of meaning and purpose to life (Averill *et al.*, 1990). It was stated by Poss (1981) earlier that where there is no hope, fear can take over, hence the importance of establishing hope for the dying patient. A terminal illness may be termed by many as a 'hopeless' situation, and it is therefore important to establish a good balance between realistic hope and acceptance of the inevitability of palliative care: this can only truly be achieved in an atmosphere of honesty and trust between the patients, their family carers and the professionals involved (Lugton, 2002). When healthcare professionals give misleading information it can prevent the patient coming to their own wrong conclusions. Alternatively, the total truth may not improve the situation, so it is important to be able to give as much of the truth, without lying,

according to what the patient and their family carers can handle, and then providing effective and appropriate support, care and treatment as required.
Good communication, understanding and dealing with the patients own fears
can help patients cope with their physical symptoms as well.

Kreiger (1982) found four phases of a terminal illness and the hopes the
patient may have during each phase.

1. In the first phase the patient hopes that there has been a mistake made with
   the diagnosis or that the illness is not palliative and will turn out to be cured.
2. With the passing of some time, the patient enters the second phase where
   hope for successful treatment predominates.
3. The third phase of hope is entered when the patient is told there is no
   further treatment which can be given to cure them. Hope is focused, then,
   on the prolongation of life.
4. Lastly, hope for a good death is the main focus, with relief from physical
   symptoms, with dignity, love and forgiveness to be shown. Hope of an afterlife may also occur, depending on the patient's own beliefs.

Lugton (2002) continues that too much information or inappropriate
information can remove a patient's hope by creating a gap between their
expectations and the reality. Too much truth about the nature of the palliative
illness can take away all hope and cause despair in the patient and their
family carers. Skilled support comes from recognising when the patient and
their carers need certain information and then by giving this in a supportive
way.

When a patient has been previously treated for cancer and either has not
entered remission for a period of time or has not responded to curative treatment, they enter the palliative stage of their illness. They may be fully aware
that their disease is no longer curative and therefore have to make huge read-
justments in their thinking from when they may have had a curative disease
to now having an incurable disease. Many such patients may feel rejected,
uncared for, unsupported, low in mood, as well as facing what the future now
brings.

In such situations it may seem silly to talk of maintaining hope. However,
although the goals of medicine and the future have changed it is still possible
to maintain hope, although it will be a very different hope to what it had been
previously.

Hope and hope-fostering strategies for patients with advanced metastatic
cancer are very important in such patients and will be different to the hope of
a fit and young, well person. The main hope will be not to suffer when imminently dying, and to live life to the fullest for the time left. Hope-fostering
strategies may include simple things such as leaving a legacy, achieving short-
term goals such as baking a cake, or getting through the day with minimal
shortness of breath, or positive thoughts, or having supportive family and
friends to help the patient through. A strong faith can be an appropriate hope-

fostering strategy for those with a strong religious or spiritual faith and can allow the patient to feel they have some control. Flemming (1997) found other hope-fostering strategies in patients in a palliative care unit, including maintaining their physical appearance and physical comfort.

When a patient is then judged not to be suitable for resuscitation, the aim is about maintaining hope when cardiopulmonary resuscitation is not an appropriate intervention. It is important to establish the difference between CPR and active treatment, as well as basic nursing care and support strategies. If a patient is not to be given, or decides not to have, CPR they must be reassured that all other care will be given. The discussion may then have to include the appropriateness of active treatments such as antibiotics, intravenous fluids, blood transfusions and so on. All of these may be appropriate in palliative care as a symptom control intervention. For example, a dying patient who develops a high temperature and agitation because of an infection may be appropriately treated with low-dose antibiotics, as well as other interventions such as paracetamol, tepid sponging or a fan, in order to help reduce the temperature, but it would need to be explained to the patient and their carers that this was a comfort intervention, not a curative treatment and to warn them that it may not actually help. Intravenous fluids may be appropriate if a terminally ill patient is unable to drink and is reporting symptomatic dehydration, such as very dry mouth and skin; however, often good, frequent mouth care works just as well. A blood transfusion may be appropriate if the patient is reporting dizziness and shortness of breath when they have a low haemoglobin count. Again, it should be emphasised to the patient and carers that this is to relieve symptoms, not a curative measure, and it does not mean that the aims of the patient's treatments have been changed.

So how can healthcare professionals maintain hope in the palliative care patient? Chaplin and McIntyre (2004) give outlines as to how to do this.

- *Comfort*: It is important to do as much to comfort the individual as possible, not only physically but psychosocially, spiritually and emotionally. Pain can be influenced by psychological, spiritual and emotional issues so if all of these are dealt with in the context of comfort then any pain experienced may be easier to assess, and for the patient to cope with.
- *Attachment*: Many palliative care patients need to be needed in the final stages of their disease. They do not wish to be rejected or forgotten, and they require caring relationships to achieve this, not only for their carers and friends but from the healthcare professionals involved in their care. This care must be given holistically.
- *Worth*: For some individuals the process of dying raises fears about their integrity and value as a person, and feelings of reduced self-worth can occur, particularly as the person who becomes less able to carry out their normal roles in life such as mother, wife, son or breadwinner.

Hope needs to be maintained in all individuals involved with patients' care, as even one person who cannot maintain hope can skew a patient's own perspectives and therefore their hope.

There may be denial in a patient and their carers which can prevent a truly good death and reduce hope. Chaplin and McIntyre (2004) suggest that this may not be true denial but a coping mechanism used by the patient and family carers in order to get through a very difficult mind shift and focus of care.

Hope is very difficult to measure since it is so subjective. Each individual will have differing levels of hope, some may appear to have no hope at all: the latter usually means that the hopes they do have are actually very unrealistic. Unrealistic hope gives way to unrealistic expectations which, when they are not achieved, can cause depression, fear, anxiety and anger. That is why it is so important when bad news is broken to the patient that not only is it truthful, but that there is no false hope or incorrect information given. It is most likely that any patients given the slightest hint of false hope will cling onto this, repeating it time again: any future news given will be measured against this hope and if the difference is much bigger than the patient was expecting it can cause depression, anger and anxiety. So, no matter how hard it may be to give bad news, and however difficult it is not to say that everything will be alright, this should never be hinted at.

Herth (1990a) designed a 12-step measurement for hope, called the 'Herth Hope Index', which has been used by healthcare professionals in terminally ill patients. There are 12 questions which the patient answers according to whether they strongly agree, agree, disagree or strongly disagree. The items on this scale can give guidance as to the specific areas of lowered hope and then specific interventions may be applied in order to try and improve any lowered areas.

Herth (1993) also carried out a longitudinal study exploring the meaning of hope in those caring for a terminally ill family member. This examined the influence of specific background characteristics on hope, and identified strategies that are used to foster hope, in a convenience sample of 25 family caregivers of terminally ill family members from two hospice programmes using the technique of methodological triangulation (interview, Herth Hope Index and Background Data Form). Hope was defined as a dynamic inner power that enables transcendence of the present situation and fosters a positive new awareness of being. Six hope-fostering categories and three hope-hindering categories were identified based on the interview responses. With the exception of those providing care to a family member diagnosed with AIDS and those caregivers experiencing poor personal health, a high fatigue level, severe sleep deprivation and more than two concurrent losses, overall hope levels among participants were found to remain stable across the background variables. Across time, hope levels were found to be low at interview time one, to rise significantly by interview time two, and then level off for the remainder of the time. An understanding of hope from the perspective of the family caregiver could provide a basis upon which to develop interventions that foster hope.

It is important that any hope is realistic (Penson, 2000), and some research by Perakyla (1991) emphasised three variations of hope work, in which the type of hope aimed for by the healthcare professional is realistic in terms of the patients' stage of disease:

- *curative hope work*: where the patient is defined as getting better
- *palliative hope work*: where the patient is defined as feeling better
- *past recovery*: where the hope is dismantled and the patient is past recovery.

The advent of the hospice movement in the 1960s heralded the recognition of this unique stage of a patient's illness trajectory and thus palliative care as a science began. With this development, and the increasing importance placed on palliative care, it is possible for patients to embrace the concept of hope not only in terminal illness and palliative care but also for those with incurable chronic diseases.

Wilkinson (1996) stated that acknowledging that cure is no longer possible does not mean that there is defeat but simply that there is now a change in perspective from dying with a terminal illness to living with one. Although it is never helpful to give false hope (in fact, it is quite the opposite) it can be useful to try and turn the patient and their family carers' aims to quality of life and aiming to help the patient live as long as possible. This does not mean length of life, and this ties in with resuscitation decisions. Aiming to keep a patient with a terminal illness, or who is imminently terminal, alive falsely by given inappropriate resuscitation does not maintain hope, even if the patient thinks it will. It will simply cause them to falsely hope for a futile end, which will be undignified and stressful. It may also cause the patient to deny how unwell they really are and thus forgo any chances of hope and realisation. Miller (1991) concluded that hope is a very important coping mechanism for those who are critically ill: it reinforces not only physiological defences but also helps patients to endure crises.

Scanlon (1989) felt that the role of the nurse was most attuned to goals of palliative medicine, since the fundamental goals of nursing are similar to those of palliative care, of alleviating suffering and providing comfort. Because nurses are also in the strategic positions to offer care they can also foster hope in order to enable the patient to live their remaining days as fully as possible (Wilkinson, 1996).

The general ethos of palliative care, and hope is included within this, should be included in all aspects of nursing. If all healthcare professionals applied the principles of palliative care in all patient care, it would ensure a more consistent, supportive, informative patient journey.

Hope is a very complex emotion but when fostered appropriately and realistically can allow a realistically acceptable quality of life and can help acceptance of eventual death.

8 The law and ethics surrounding resuscitation

Certain aspects of the law and ethics relating to resuscitation have already been mentioned briefly. This chapter will now discuss some of these legal and ethical issues pertaining to resuscitation in more detail, such as euthanasia, Advance Directives and Human Rights, in order to enhance the reader's knowledge and confidence in such matters. These subjects have a huge amount of literature already written, so further information can easily be gleaned from other sources, if the reader wishes.

Tschudin (1992) states the word *ethics* actually comes from the greek word *eros* meaning 'character', whereas *morals* comes from the Latin for 'custom' or 'manner', that is, fundamental ways of conduct which are not only customary but right.

Bioethics (ethics relating to healthcare professions) came into being as its own discipline in the 1970s. As medical technology has advanced so has the need for bioethics in order to offer some control and advice to those involved with decision-making in the healthcare professions. Bioethics can give order to the relationships and treatments offered to patients. Patients build relationships with healthcare professionals in order for the appropriate outcomes to their care to be achieved. These relationships are a kind of agreement between the patient and the professionals, and ethics can help to order this agreement and protect those involved in it, in particular the patient. Certain ethics are lead by the ethical codes of either deontology or utilitarianism. On the face of it, these can be quite complicated but they may be simplified.

DEONTOLOGY

This ethical code makes 'right' and 'wrong' the central concepts. It involves doing one's duty and doing what is right. To not do this means the individual has shirked their duty. Beyond actually doing the right thing and not doing the wrong thing, there is little else involved in this ethical code. The outcome of the action taken is not relevant, whether it is what was wanted or what was not. According to deontological theory a person is not morally responsible for the results of their action, only for the action itself. Doing one's duty is central to this code. Deontology demands actions without regard for consequences. Immanuel Kant (1724–1804) was the most powerful leader of this code and he felt that a person was born knowing their duty. Unfortunately, this code would be very difficult to justify in the modern day medical world. Medical staff must think of the consequences of their actions, and should be able to justify their actions and interventions. A nurse cannot justify her actions by saying, 'I was doing my duty'. Thus resuscitation decisions under this code would be decided according to what was right for the patient but with no regard to the outcome. As such decisions are mainly based on whether resuscitation would be successful or futile, the outcome of the action, this code would not really help in resuscitation decisions.

UTILITARIANISM

The central concepts in this code which is sometimes referred to as 'consequentialism' are of 'good' and 'evil'. Its basis is in hedonism, which states all actions ought to be motivated by pleasure and pain. Determinism, as well as hedonism, is the drive for this code and it states that every human action is a response to a prior drive. Thus choice and decision-making are illusions. People cannot escape viewing pleasure as the 'good'. The good of two people is the greater good, and thus the greatest good for the majority of people is the goal of every ethical agent. However, under this code it would be difficult for a healthcare professional to justify their actions by the utilitarianism code of 'the greatest good for the greatest number'. The professional's principal responsibility is to the individual patient, and that patient, in turn, has a right to choose their own goals and decide their own consequences, where possible. If the utilitarian code was followed, the nurse would have no time for individualised patient care and the patient would have no right to expect individualised care. This ethical code is further split into 'act utilitarianism', which concentrates on the act itself required to give the greatest good to the greatest number, and 'rule utilitarianism', which states that a rule is right if it provides the greatest outcome for the greatest number. In terms of resuscitation decisions this ethical code would not be helpful either, as it would look at what was right for the most patients, not on an individual basis. As said before, each resuscitation decision must be individualised and cannot be decided upon simply because of age or diagnosis.

   Other ethical codes are provided for doctors and nurses by the professional bodies they subscribe to, for example, the Nursing and Midwifery Council (NMC) *Code of Professional Conduct* (NMC 2004) provides a list of clauses for the conduct of all nurses, midwives and health visitors, both towards their own colleagues and to patients. However, Singleton and McLaren (1995) argue that such a list of clauses can be a little ambiguous. For example, one of the clauses in the nurses *Code* states that nurses should act in the 'patient's interests', to maintain their 'well-being', and their 'safety'. Singleton and McLaren (1995) argue that these terms are subjective and not clear-cut, particularly in the multi-cultural societies in which care is now given. Thus, care in healthcare settings may not be as clear-cut, even when given according to certain ethical codes and guidelines, as perhaps it could be.

Ethics is concerned with 'actions taken in the pursuit of vital and fundamental goals'. The ethical aspects of a given situation are determined by what is important in that situation. What is important in that situation is what is determined by the purposes of the individuals who can act in it. The nurse or healthcare professional must be concerned with the appropriateness of their purposes and the foreseeable ethical outcomes of the actions they take. But how does a healthcare professional know what are truly appropriate actions and purposes? This knowledge tends to come through experience and learning, something which is very difficult to do by reading or studying alone. The patient is the agent of the nurse, and every ethical decision a nurse makes, as a nurse, must hold the patient as the central focus. Thus the first important step in any ethical decision-making is to make the patient the most important aspect and to think of foreseeable outcomes in terms of how it will affect the patient.

In order for any healthcare professional to be able to act individually in ethical decision-making there needs to be certain ethical interactions between the patient and the healthcare worker. The main understanding in ethical interaction is that the patient has rights that will not be violated. These rights are governed through ethical standards, or principles. As Western society has become more conscious of the complexity of moral problems, ethical decisions have strayed from the implicit domain of the medical and clerical professionals. In the 1980s these ethical principles emerged for use in ethical decision-making, particularly in medicine (Beauchamp and Childress, 2001):

- *Beneficence*: Doing good, contributing to a person's welfare. This means the doctors caring for the patient are obliged to act in the best interests of the patient by weighing up the benefits versus the side effects. Beneficence takes more positive steps to help someone rather than just passively not inflicting harm which is the second principle.
- *Non-maleficence*: Not inflicting harm. This is related to the medical principle of *Primum non noce* (Above all, do no harm). This means the doctors are obliged to do no harm, and this principle may be failed at the end of life when certain doctors may be worried about given analgesics or sedatives to a patient who is clearly in distress, because they are concerned about hastening death.
- *Respect for autonomy*: The choices of individuals must be respected. An autonomous individual is one who has the right and power to take action according to personal desire and without obtaining permission. Autonomy

is an individual's 'moral property' and is concerned with the uniqueness of that individual, and with protecting that uniqueness. Autonomy is related to informed consent, which allows a reasonable person to make autonomous decisions regarding treatment choices (Rousseau, 2001) but only when those treatment choices are possible. Respect for patient autonomy, as seen before, is not an absolute ethical principle. However, although autonomy takes precedence when the patient disagrees with the doctor, it does not follow that the patient can demand or insist they are given certain treatments which may be harmful or inappropriate. This ethical principle may conflict with the fourth principle of justice.

- *Justice*: This means that doctors are obliged to treat similar patients with similar problems with the same interventions. Thus, resources must be shared across society equally. There should be fairness in treatments offered according to what the patient is entitled to.
- *Freedom*: An individual can possess freedom without making an agreement but they cannot make an agreement without possessing freedom. This principle means that the patient has freedom to make their own decisions and a freedom to have their rights acknowledged and respected.
- *Veracity*: This literally means truthfulness. There must be confidence in the veracity of those involved in any agreement, both from the side of the healthcare professional and the patient. If this does not exist it is impossible for true decision-making to take place since there will be no regard or respect from all parties involved.
- *Privacy*: This is the right of the individual to be free of undesired interactions or relationships and the healthcare professional has an obligation to protect her patient from undesirable interactions. A patient does give up a part of their privacy to the healthcare professional but does not need to give up all of it. Part of privacy includes confidentiality which the healthcare worker must maintain in all the patient's affairs.

In resuscitation beneficence should be taken into account as to whether the actual act of resuscitation will be possibly successful or futile. Non-maleficence should be considered in terms of whether resuscitation will cause harm because it is futile. Respect for autonomy means listening to the patient's own views about resuscitation. Although this can conflict with futility and although the medical opinion may be not to resuscitate, part of the resuscitation discussion can include whether the patient is shocked or upset by the news that they will not be resuscitated, and then move on and explain the rationale behind the DNAR order. In this way the patient is able to express their concerns, or agreement, and can feel part of the decision-making process even when they may not really have been. If there is a chance of success from resuscitation, and the patient is adamant they wish to be resuscitated, then such a decision can be made with their consent: a patient has a right to be resuscitated if the procedure is likely to be successful (Dimond, 2004). It is possible that a patient may have a high chance of success (though not if they are imminently terminal or have widespread metastatic disease) but may not wish to be resuscitated anyway. Justice can include not only what is right to treat the patient with physically, but also in terms of resource allocation and cost-effectiveness (Edwards, 1996). Although ethically cost cannot be the only reason why resuscitation is not carried out it is certainly considered to be a factor in futility. Freedom means the individual has rights which should be respected. In this way, in terms of resuscitation decisions, their rights include being allowed to be told the truth and to be aware of what their treatment would, and would not, include. Veracity links into freedom in that the doctors would be honest with the patient and explain the likelihood of resuscitation being successful; the patient would respect this decision because of the honesty and truthfulness given to them, and because the doctor respected their need to know the truth if they wanted. Privacy means the patient may not want to be involved in decision-making and this should be acceptable: but they would need to be aware of having a choice, which should be respected. The patient's confidentiality would be maintained through this, and thus the patient would be consulted first, not the family carers. Personal information to do with their health and care should only be shared with others if the patient agrees to this.

There can be ethical conflict between the principles of autonomy, beneficence and non-maleficence, if a patient wants resuscitation but the doctor thinks it will be futile. The NCPC (2003) states that there is no ethical obligation to discuss such a decision. However, if truth-telling is to be obeyed, such a decision and its rationale should be explained to the patient.

To resuscitate when a decision has been made not to can be seen as assault and to not resuscitate someone who is for resuscitation can be seen as negligence and can be subject to criminal charges (Dimond, 2002). There are certain situations where using only one ethical standard therefore may not be particularly helpful. In these circumstances it would be appropriate to make decisions without using these ethical standards implicitly. However, there would still need to be tacit understanding and agreement that the individual be respected for their uniqueness, and that no harm be done to that patient deliberately.

The ethical code of deontology conflicts with the ethical standards listed above.

* Deontology conflicts with autonomy because it does not look at individualised patient care and is not a code which promotes a person's happiness: personal choice is not included, simply doing the right thing. The healthcare professional's actions and decisions would be irrelevant to the patient. What counts is the moral quality of those decisions and actions.
* Deontology conflicts with freedom because it demands only doing what is right and not what is wrong. It takes no account for the patient's own individual choices and rights.

- Deontology conflicts with veracity because truth is not a value through which human purposes are attained in deontology. Doing what is right is the only driving force; there is no room for individual needs or choices.
- Deontology conflicts with beneficence because the duty of deontology is to do what is right and it does not take into account whether good or whether harm will be done to the patient. If good is done, this is only an outcome from what is done; it was not the reason *why* the action was carried out.

The ethical code of utilitarianism conflicts with ethical standards as well.

- Utilitarianism conflicts with autonomy because there is no place for individual needs or concerns. Utilitarianism is concerned with the greatest good for the greatest number.
- Utilitarianism conflicts with freedom, again because of there being no room for individual concerns or respect for individual's needs and choices. In the case of the healthcare professional they would use paternalism instead.
- Utilitarianism conflicts with veracity because the utilitarianist must ignore truth and do what is best for the greatest number of patients.
- Utilitarianism conflicts with privacy because the patient's right to privacy would be ignored in order to gain the best for the largest number of people. The individual would not be of importance.
- Utilitarianism conflicts with beneficence because the outcome of a decision or action on the individual is not important: it is the best outcome for the largest number which is the driving force.

POWER OF ATTORNEY

There is nothing legal in England, Wales or Northern Ireland for relatives to make any medical decisions by proxy, even if given Power of Attorney. However, their opinion of the patient's own views may be useful. Those with Durable Power of Attorney can decide on financial and property affairs, even if the donor (i.e. the person for whom they have Power of Attorney) becomes mentally unstable. Ordinary Power of Attorney is not valid for these affairs if the person becomes mentally unstable. Note that this only applies to financial and property affairs, not medical decisions. Scotland has the Welfare Power of Attorney whereby the person *can* make medical decisions for the donor.

Under English law, adults deemed of sound mind can refuse or consent to be examined or treated, even if it is life-saving (Birtwhistle and Nielson, 1998).

ADVANCE DIRECTIVES

Advance directives (Living Wills) are now legally recognised in this country by Common Law but there is no act of Parliament setting out the law. The document, if signed and witnessed, allows a person to set out what they want to happen to them in the event of them being incapacitated and requiring resuscitation or any other treatment, as long as it has been witnessed correctly and the person was deemed of sound mind when it was made (BMA *et al.*, 2001). The doctor, if he sees the document to represent the wishes of the patient, can use it as a defence to any actions taken because of it.

Beauchamp and Childress (2001) argue that such Advance Directives made and witnessed appropriately can be helpful in decision-making for the family and reduce stress on them and healthcare professionals during a stressful time. They can, however, raise some practical and ethical problems:

• they are often not very explicit
• the patient may have changed their mind between making the Advance Directive and the time when a decision needs to be made (however, Neuberger (2004) says that as long as such directives are updated every three to five years, this issue would not become a problem)
• some patients may not fully understand all the implications of what they are signing, or realise what advancing medical technology may now be able to achieve.

Advance Directives, however, do not accomplish their aims and this may apply to resuscitation decisions. Regardless of this, many people are very keen to make one in order to try and make sure their wishes are known and understood if they are unable to voice them personally.

There is no rule in Great Britain for decision-making by proxy, and advance directives are now legally recognised; however, if there is any doubt as to whether the patient still agrees with their Advance Directive decision the advice of their family carers should be sought.

HUMAN RIGHTS ACT 1998

The UK was a signatory of the European Convention for the Protection of Human Rights and Fundamental Freedoms 1953. However, anyone trying to bring action against a breach of human rights, as set out in this convention, was not actually able to take the case to court in this country but had to go to the European Court of Human Rights in Strasbourg. This was a lengthy and expensive process, which could take up to five years and cost as much as £30,000. As expected, because of this, few cases ever came to light. However, with the Human Rights Act of 1998 coming into effect in October 2000 an allegation of a breach of human rights can be brought to courts in England. It is now also illegal for a public authority to breach the rights set out in the original Convention, and judges can now declare that legislation brought before them which is in breach of the Convention can be sent back to Parliament to be altered.

There are certain rights listed in the Convention and two of these main articles relate mostly to medical care and resuscitation.

- The Right to Life (Article 2(1)) states: 'Everyone's right to life shall be protected by law. No one shall be deprived of his life intentionally save in the execution of a sentence of a court following his conviction for which this penalty is provided by law.'

Dimond (2002) states that this article has been used when a person has been refused treatment or resuscitation, or treatment is withdrawn or withheld. However, such cases are examined in terms of the person's medical status and in terms of other articles in the Human Rights Act. For example, the parents of a disabled baby wanted the doctors' decision for DNAR to be overruled, but it was decided that this did not contravene Article 2 and that a dignified approach to the baby's last few weeks was the most appropriate. Therefore in the cases of patients deemed inappropriate for resuscitation, as long as the rationale is appropriate, this would not be against the Human Rights Act.

- The Right Not to be Subjected to Inhuman or Degrading Treatment (Article 3) states: 'No one shall be subjected to torture or to inhuman or degrading treatment or punishment'.

It may be argued that the care administered in certain hospitals, nursing or care homes and when patients lay on stretchers in A+E for many hours, could be interpreted as inhuman and degrading treatment. It can also be argued that resuscitating someone when it is inappropriate could contravene this article.

These human rights tie in with the ethical principles of beneficence and non-maleficence because these rights state that no one should be subjected to inhuman treatment (of which inappropriate cardiopulmonary resuscitation (CPR) could be seen as) or to not have appropriate treatment (i.e. being made DNAR when success rates are high in that patient's physical condition).

DOCUMENTATION

All resuscitation decisions need to be documented in the medical notes, or on an appropriate form which is filed in the patient's medical notes, and communicated to all those caring for that patient. Dimond (2002) further states that when a DNAR order is made that everyone on the team understands the rationale behind the decision. She also states that it cannot be a verbal order but must be written down to make it a legal statement. She states that the only reasons not to resuscitate are the ones listed in the resuscitation guidelines:

- the mentally competent patient has refused treatment
- a valid Living Will (Advance Directive) covering such circumstances has been made by the competent person

- effective cardiopulmonary resuscitation is unlikely to be successful;
- where successful resuscitation is likely to be followed by a length and quality of life that would not be in the best interests of the patient to sustain.

Dimond (2002) argues it is still appropriate to discuss with patients what their views might be where a resuscitation decision is not clear-cut, in order to explore their wishes.

WITHHOLDING OR WITHDRAWING TREATMENT

Rousseau (2000) believes that there is no difference between withholding or withdrawing treatment, that in fact they are one and the same thing. This is because carrying out either for a person who is able to speak for themselves and requests this is permissible and if they are unable to vocalise their wishes then the views of the family carers as to what the patient would have wanted, are able to be sought. He continues that the decision to withhold or withdraw treatments is based on four things:

- the patient's wishes
- medical indications
- benefits and burdens of treatment
- quality of life that may result from the treatment.

It is actually easier not to start a treatment that the doctor thinks may not be helpful than to start it and later need to stop it. This can cause confusion and distress for the patient and their family carers, and even for other healthcare professionals caring for that patient.

The British Medical Associaton (BMA) (2002) stated, in its guidance on withholding or withdrawing treatment, that:

End of natural life:

Life has a natural end, and doctors and others caring for a patient need to recognise that the point may come in the progression of a patient's condition where death is drawing near. In these circumstances doctors should not strive to prolong the dying process with no regard to the patient's wishes, where known, or an up to date assessment of the benefits and burdens of treatment or non-treatment.

Care for the dying:

Patients who are dying should be afforded the same respect and standard of care as all other patients. Patients and their families and others close to them should be treated with understanding and compassion. Where the likely progression of a patient's condition is known, and their death is seen as an inevitable outcome, it is important to ensure that the patient's palliative care or terminal care needs are identified and met appropriately. This should include consideration of their wishes regarding such matters as the appropriate place for receiving care (which may affect the treatment options available), and their needs for religious, spiritual or other personal support. Every attempt should be made to ensure that they are afforded privacy, dignity, and good quality care in comfortable surroundings. This includes assessment of, and adequate relief from, pain and other distressing symptoms, and appropriate support and nursing care.

Discussion about the dying process allows patients the opportunity they may want to decide what arrangements should be made to manage the final stages of their illness, and to attend to personal and other concerns that they consider important towards the end of their life.

The BMA suggest further consideration on the following:

- Whether respect for human life means doctors have to offer all means in order to prolong life.
- Would it be unlawful?
- Who should be involved in the decision? Whose views have weight?

The document (BMA, 2002) continues by saying there should also be an obligation to work within the law and that life has a natural end which patients, carers and healthcare workers all need to recognise. Whatever decision is thus made must be committed to by all those caring for the patient, including the patient and family carers, and accurately recorded and regularly reviewed (See also UKCC, 1998). If not everyone is aware of such a decision it could cause further distress. Doctors should take patients' views into account but the BMA (2002) argue that doctors have no ethical obligation to offer a treatment which is deemed to be futile.

These statements further clarify that anyone who has a poor prognosis or poor quality of life needs good palliative care, and that, legally, treatment and resuscitation can be withdrawn as long as the rationale behind the decisions is sound.

A DNAR order could be interpreted by some as withholding a treatment. However, Beauchamp and Childress (2001) and Randall (2003) argue that if a patient is dying and CPR is seen as futile, it is imperative to prevent harm to the patient and thus make a DNAR decision. Randall (2003) takes this further by stating that such a decision is justified, regardless of the patient's and family carers' wishes.

EUTHANASIA

Tschudin (1992) states the definitions of euthanasia.

- *Voluntary*: When a patient's life is ended by another with the patient's consent.
- *Active*: When a patient's life is ended by another without the patient's consent.
- *Passive*: The ending of someone's life by withholding helpful treatment at the patient's request.

- *Involuntary*: The ending of someone's life by withholding helpful treatment without patient's request.

Euthanasia is not recognised by law in the UK. In law it is recognised that there is a difference between letting someone die and killing a person. Withdrawing inappropriate treatment is seen as letting someone die. This is very different from deliberately giving medications or treatment which will speed this process up. Since 1961 suicide has not been a crime. However much a person or member of staff may sympathise with someone's wish to die they are prohibited by criminal law in assisting in giving any help or advice for the patient to be able to carry out their wish.

Family carers of the patient may talk of the patient suffering when that person is near death. They may talk of the fact that a dog or animal in a similar situation would be 'put down' (Neuberger, 2004). It is clear from this that the family carers are finding it hard to watch their relative die. However, legally, the best way forward in this situation is to reassure them and make sure that good palliative care is more appropriate to help prevent as much suffering for the patient as possible, which may in turn help the family carers to accept this situation more readily. It is because of the sanctity of life in Western culture that euthanasia has not yet been legalised in this country.

Neuberger (2004) argues that the issue of euthanasia is complicated further in Britain by the cost of full-time care for those unable to care for themselves any longer. The cost of nursing homes for those older people who can no longer look after themselves means that their house, or inheritance money, is often eaten up by the fees for the home, leaving families with less, or nothing, in terms of inheritance money. Many families will not really see this as an issue, but others unfortunately do. They may feel it is a right that they should inherit something, that their parents would have wanted them to have the money. They may actually have committed themselves financially to something with the idea that the inheritance money will help them out of a sticky situation, or will enable them to achieve something they have always wanted, such as a luxury house or money to invest in a new business. These families may see euthanasia as a way of preventing the loss of possibly such a huge amount of money. This has meant that the laws against euthanasia need to be very strictly adhered to as many people are worried about euthanasia being used for the wrong reasons.

Concern has been expressed by some nursing and medical staff that giving 'as required' (prn) medication (e.g. diamorphine) to someone who is dying may 'speed up' the process, and that this action would not be seen as legal. An interpretation of such an action is the 'Doctrine of Double Effect' (DDE). As long as the drug was given for the right reasons, such as the patient was in pain, very agitated, or very breathless, this action would be interpreted as double effect if the patient died soon afterwards.

PASSIVE EUTHANASIA

It has been suggested that not resuscitating someone could be interpreted as passive euthanasia, that is, euthanasia occurring through non-treatment. However, in view of the previous paragraph and arguments expressed, treatment is not always appropriate and, if a DNAR order has been made with the appropriate rationale, such a death is not passive euthanasia. Everyone will have to die one day.

Beauchamp and Childress (2001) argued that making a patient a DNAR order without that person's consent could therefore be seen as passive euthanasia, but only if the CPR *would be seen as successful for that person*. Looking at the definitions of euthanasia above, DNAR in someone where it is deemed to be futile does not come under passive euthanasia because resuscitation in this case is not seen to be helpful.

Beauchamp and Childress (2001) also discuss the difference between killing someone and letting someone die. Killing is a causal action that brings about death, whereas letting someone die is intentional avoidance of causal interventions so that disease, system failure or injury causes death. In medical terms, letting someone die can be acceptable if a medical technology is futile, or if a patient has validly refused a medical technology. Thus letting a patient die by making them a DNAR order if resuscitation is deemed futile, or if a patient refuses resuscitation, is acceptable. At this point, good patient care and support to them and their family carers is important (Tschudin, 1992).

THE RIGHT TO DIE A 'GOOD DEATH'

Tschudin (1992) links this debate in with the one on euthanasia. Most people agree that dying with dignity is preferable to lingering and suffering. The opposite of euthanasia must be good care of dying patients, that is, good palliative care. This does not mean the patient is abandoned to die without care.

THE DOCTRINE OF DOUBLE EFFECT

This principle was developed in the Middle Ages by the Roman Catholic moral theologians, and is used in ethical and moral situations. The Doctrine states that if doing something morally good has a morally bad outcome it is ethically acceptable to do the act providing the bad outcome was not intentional. This is true even if the bad outcome was known to possibly occur and foreseen. Under this Doctrine, an action is permissible if the act is good or morally neutral; the good effect is the intent of the practitioner; the good effect is not achieved through the bad effect; and that there is a proportionately grave reason for undertaking the action or, in other words, the good effect must exceed the bad effect.

This principle is used to justify the case where a doctor or nurse gives drugs, such as analgesics or sedatives, to a terminally ill patient in order to relieve distressing symptoms, even though the doctor or nurse is aware that the action of doing this may shorten the patient's life (Cherny *et al.*, 1994; Mayo, 1996; Rousseau, 2000). In this circumstance the Doctrine is honoured, negating any suggestion that the action was inappropriate on the part of the healthcare professional. This is because the aim of the action is not directly to kill the patient – the bad result of the patient's death is a *side-effect* of the good intention, that of reducing the patient's pain or other symptoms. There should be an appropriate dose of drugs given, which is therapeutic but takes into account whether the patient is already on the medication. For instance, a patient who has never had morphine before but is in pain is first given a small, appropriate dose of morphine. However, if a patient has been on a high dose of morphine but still has pain the dose given for any breakthrough pain would be a one-sixth of the total daily dose of morphine (Twycross and Wilcock, 2002) as too small a dose would not have an effect.

Many healthcare professionals use this doctrine to justify the use of high doses of drugs such as morphine for the purpose of relieving suffering in terminally ill patients, even though they know the drugs are likely to cause the patient to die sooner. The BBC website has some helpful information on this doctrine.

Factors involved in the Doctrine of Double Effect:

- The good result must be achieved independently of the bad one.
- For the doctrine to apply, the bad result must not be the means of achieving the good one. So if the only way the drug relieves the patient's pain is by killing them, the Doctrine of Double effect doesn't apply.
- The action must be proportional to the cause. If a patient were given a dose of drugs so large that it is certain to kill them, and that is also far greater than the dose needed to control their pain, the Doctrine of Double Effect could not be applied.
- The action must be appropriate. The right medicine must be given for the right symptom/problem. If the patient were given a fatal dose of pain-killing drugs, it's no use saying that the intention was to relieve their symptoms of vomiting if the drug doesn't have any effect on vomiting.
- The action must be appropriate. The patient needs the right medicine for their symptoms. If the patient is given a fatal dose of pain-killing drugs, it's no use saying that the intention was to relieve their symptoms of pain if the patient wasn't suffering from pain but from breathlessness.
- The patient must be in a terminal condition. If a fatal dose of pain-killing drugs is administered and the patient would have recovered from their disease or injury if it hadn't been given it's no use saying that the intention was to relieve

their pain. And that applies even if there was no other way of controlling their pain.

Problems with the Doctrine of Double Effect

Some philosophers think this argument is too clever for its own good.

- We are responsible for all the anticipated consequences of our actions
- If the two effects of the action can be foreseen there is a moral responsibility for both effects.
- Intention is irrelevant. Some people take the view that it's sloppy morality to decide the rightness or wrongness of an act by looking at the intention of the doctor. They think that some acts are objectively right or wrong, and that the intention of the person who does them is irrelevant. But most legal systems regard the intention of a person as a vital element in deciding whether they have committed a crime, and how serious a crime, in cases of causing death.
- Death is not always bad – so double effect is irrelevant. Other philosophers say that the Doctrine of Double Effect assumes that death is always bad. They say that if continued life holds nothing for the patient but the negative things of pain and suffering, then death is a good thing, and the doctrine of double effect is not needed.
- Double effect can produce an unexpected moral result. If a quicker death is seen as better than a slower one then the Doctrine of Double Effect shows that a doctor who intended to kill the patient is morally superior to a doctor who merely intended to relieve pain.

The Sulmasy test

Daniel P Sulmasy has put forward a way for a doctor or nurse to check their intention in carrying out an intervention or treatment. The doctor should ask himself, 'If the patient were not to die after my actions, would I feel that I had failed to accomplish what I had set out to do?'.

Beauchamp and Childress (2001) describe the doctrine of double effect as, 'a single act having two foreseen effects, one good and one harmful'. In palliative care an example of this is the giving of an analgesic to a dying patient who is in pain. If a doctor or nurse gives something to intentionally kill them, this act is actually murder. However, if they give something for pain relief at an acceptable dose, but the patient quickly deteriorates and dies then this is acceptable because the intention of giving the analgesic was good. There are four elements to the doctrine of double effect described (Beauchamp and Childress, 2001):

- the nature of the act: the act must be good in itself
- *intention*: this must be for good effect; the bad effect may be noted but must not be intended
- distinction between means and effects: the bad effect must be means to the good effect. If the good effect was the result of the bad effect the person doing the act would intend the bad effect in pursuit of the good.
- the good effect must outweigh the bad: the bad effect is permissible only if a proportionate reason compensates for permitting the foreseen bad effect.

Craig (2002) highlights the possible dangers of terminal sedation without hydration. She shows how advocates of euthanasia in the UK and elsewhere are exploiting the practice of 'terminal sedation' and how the ethical and legal risks of sedation in palliative care would be reduced if carers took a more active approach to hydration.

Sedation when given with the sole intention of relieving suffering at the end of life has become acceptable practice, but Craig (2002) feels this is a highly controversial subject in palliative care. She has felt previously (Craig, 1994) that such sedation could actually be used by the supporters of euthanasia as a legal means to ending life more quickly in those who are imminently terminal. The practice of terminal sedation is called 'slow euthanasia' (a phrase coined by Billings and Block, 1996), by those who want to advocate for euthanasia themselves.

Dr Michael Irwin a prominent member of the Voluntary Euthanasia Society, has stated (Irwin, 2001) that slow euthanasia is widely used in hospitals, hospices and nursing homes, whereby a doctor may legally prescribe increasing doses of regular analgesics and sedative drugs in a legal way according to known guidelines, policies and protocols, and achieve euthanasia legally, as long as the medication is used to relieve a person's suffering at the end of life. According to Irwin (2001), 70 doctors signed the 'Boston Declaration on Assisted Dying', at the biannual World Federation of Right-To-Die Societies, held in USA in September 2000. This declaration states in one paragraph:

> A physician may lawfully administer increasing doses of regular analgesic and sedative drugs that can hasten someone's death as long as the declared intent is to ease the pain and suffering . . . Compassionate physicians, without publicly declaring the true intention of their actions, often speed up the dying process in this way. Many thousands of terminally ill patients are so helped globally every year . . . as it is totally uncontrolled this procedure is open to abuse.

Craig (2002) states that although the allegations in the Boston Declaration are serious they would be difficult to substantiate, as when a patient is dying it is hard to prove, beyond reasonable doubt, that life was shortened by the treatment given. The fact that euthanasia is illegal in this country makes any reliable information impossible to obtain (Tumim Committee, 2001).

The subject of evidence for hydration and sedation has little research. Quill *et al.* (1997) stated that terminal sedation alongside the voluntary stopping of eating and drinking was closer to physician-assisted suicide and voluntary active euthanasia. This paper caused outcry amongst many healthcare professionals.

Craig (2002) found that doctors use different levels of intervention depending on things such as stoism and the wishes of the patient. Some patients, if given a choice, may prefer not to have sedation, whereas others who may be very frightened of dying would rather be sedated. Irwin (2001) also states that the differences in choices of sedation and how much intervention is given tends to be consistent according to the hospital or medical centre and therefore according to certain doctors and not necessarily patient need. Craig (2002), however, does appreciate that when sedation is used appropriately it can give relief to terminally agitated patients, but that each situation should be approached sensitively and according to patient need, not doctor's standard procedures.

Thorns and Sykes (2000), on a retrospective study of 238 consecutive hospice patients, stated that, 'Appropriate use of opioids does not shorten life and there is little if any need to invoke DDE' (DDE stands for doctrine of double effect) and the authors found little difference between those patients who had a marked increased in opioid doses in their last week of life compared to those who did not. These authors stated as well that, 'The DDE may be a useful principle that can offer reassurance to healthcare professionals facing difficult treatment decisions, but it must be distinguished from euthanasia, and its role should not be exaggerated.'

Sedation is widely used in end-of life care, but little has been published about the link between sedation and hydration. Irwin (2001) stated that terminal sedation amounts to euthanasia 'because the comatose patient often dies from the combination of two intentional acts by a doctor: the induction of unconsciousness and the withholding of fluid and water. And so, for many, terminal sedation is really society's wink to euthanasia, for on the surface it looks like a combination of accepted practices of aggressive comfort care and the withdrawal of life-sustaining treatment', and states that such sedation means palliative care practitioners can argue they are keeping the palliative patient in a pharmacologically induced coma rather than deal with the fact that they may be ending someone's life.

Craig (2002), however, does share the views that prolonged use of sedation without hydration is tantamount to euthanasia, and that the hospice movement has been very slow to grasp this concept and accept how useful hydration is for patient comfort and safety. Billings (1995) actually advocates the use of sedation without hydration in the patient who is experiencing intractable suffering.

All palliative care workers with experience will have their own views on this. Each situation needs to be individually assessed. However, the professional cannot forever hide behind the curtain of the Doctrine of Double Effect. Yes, as long as the intention of the action is for the good that is fine. However, the use of hydration must, as all of the actions of healthcare professionals, be based on sound knowledge where possible and good clinical judgement.

A DNAR decision, if made because resuscitation is deemed to be futile, is good, as it has good intentions. Yes, the bad effect is that the patient will die but they will, it is hoped, die with dignity and peacefully.

INFORMED CONSENT AND RESUSCITATION

Beauchamp and Childress (2001) state that the term of 'informed consent' first occurred in the late 1950s but received attention properly from the 1970s. They state that there have been changes in what should be included in consent recently, so that not only is the patient consenting to a treatment but is also understanding the procedure and possible complications. The intention of informed consent is to protect the patient's autonomous choice, and such consent is an individual's autonomous authorisation of a medical intervention or of participation in research. Beauchamp and Childress (2001) give elements which should be included in informed consent:

- competence to understand and decide
- disclosure of material information
- understanding of the disclosure
- voluntariness in the decision
- consent itself.

In resuscitation decisions some of these elements must be included in order to explain the rationale. However, voluntariness and consent are not required in order for a decision to be made, because of the elements of success. CPR is one of the only decisions in medicine for which it is decided *not* to be given. All other treatments are for if the treatment *should* be given.

Can informed consent ever truly be informed? It surely relies on how much information is given, and also on the teaching and learning techniques which the giver and receiver have. Often, patients do not understand but are too intimidated or unwell to ask further questions. Culture, belief systems and language issues may also skew understanding of the information given. For these reasons it may be argued that true informed consent is never possible. Edwards (1996) states that it is evident that knowledge of specific information is necessary for a person for make a competent decision. 'Relevant information' depends on the giver's interpretation and own knowledge.

CONFIDENTIALITY

Legally, morally and professionally there is strong justification for confidentiality for both verbal and written records of patient care. This confidentiality applies to anything to do with patient care, and anything to do with the healthcare work, such as budgets and staffing. The BMA is clear as to what may be breached in terms of patient records and in what exceptional circumstances. However, the World Health Organization feels that there is an absolute duty of care to the patient which continues even after they have died. For nurses, the *Code of Professional Conduct* (NMC, 2004) states that confidentiality shall be respected except when disclosure is required by law, or when the patient agrees it, or when it is in their or someone else's interests. The same applies for documentation of resuscitation or of anything else to do with that patient: it is confidential and only those who need to know this, such as healthcare workers involved with that patient, should know it. If the patient chooses to tell everyone in their bay, that is up to them. However, if such information seems to distress certain other patients, that patient may need to be told to be a little less effusive with their information. What healthcare workers need to be aware of is their duty of care to that patient. If confidentialities are broken then so will be the patient's trust and relationship with that professional.

FAMILY AND PATIENT CONFLICT IN RESUSCITATION DECISIONS

This has already been discussed in Chapter 4. The failing of many doctors is to inform or ask the relatives about CPR decisions without discussing with the competent patient. The decision is then made without discussion with the patient, who may not even be told the outcome. Many relatives then request such a decision is not made evident to the patient. This is often because they do not want their relative to be upset. If the patient is told first this solves the problem. However, if the family ask that a patient not be told anything if there are any decisions to be made, or to be told any bad news, this needs to be resolved according to Peter Kaye's (1996) methods (as discussed in Chapter 4).

JUSTIFIED STRONG MEDICAL PATERNALISM

Medical paternalism has been seen in a rather negative way previously. Paternalism can be defined as: 'a refusal to accept or to acquiesce in another person's wishes, choices or actions, for that person's benefit' (Childress, 1982). It describes treating the patient almost as an adult would treat a child, or when the healthcare worker (in this case the doctor) assumes the authority of a parent. It does not take into account the patient's own rights, values and beliefs. Historically, paternalism was associated with the patient as a passive person. However, Beauchamp and Childress (2001) argue that it can actually be justified. For example, if a doctor decides a patient is inappropriate to have resuscitation because it would be futile, and even though the patient may not agree with the decision made, this is justifiable if such an action will spare the dying patient and their family carers' pointless grief and suffering.

Beauchamp and Childress (2001) continue to argue that strong medical paternalism is acceptable if:

- a patient is at risk of significant, presumable harm
- the paternalistic action will prevent harm
- the projected benefits to the patient of the paternalistic action outweigh its risks to the patient
- the least autonomy-restrictive alternative that will secure the benefits and reduce the risks is adopted (e.g. active treatment).

With the rise of consumerism, human rights and equal opportunities, paternalism has shifted so that now the patient's rights are emphasised, ensuring that patients are given a choice where there is one.

QUALITY OF LIFE VERSUS SANCTITY OF LIFE

Thiroux (1980) states that, 'Human beings should revere life and accept death'. In order for the sanctity of life to be fully understood there must be a good understanding of what is meant by 'life'. The meaning of what life is includes its physiological processes and how they interact; the basic needs required in order to survive (water, food, air, shelter, companionship); consciousness, thoughts and emotions, and memory; the value of various activities, such as socialising, walking, working and physical self-expression. If this is life, what is death? Rachels (1986) defines it in terms of biological life and biographical life, that is, not just being alive in terms of breathing, eating, *being* live, but also in terms of being able to liaise with other living beings and having a concept of being alive. Thus, Rachels' (1986) view would mean that those in a persistent vegetative state would not be truly alive as they would not be interacting with other live beings. He states this by saying: 'this means that "brain death" precludes any restoration of consciousness: at that point we can be sure that the donor's organs are no longer of any use to him. So it is morally right to fix the time of death at that point' (Rachels, 1986, p. 43). All these things need to be recognised when determining the sanctity of life itself. Life is also the precondition of all values, since nothing can be desired or sought by anyone unless they are alive. 'No one can desire to be happy, to act well, and live well, who does not at the same time desire to be, to act, and to live, that is to say, actually to exist' (Benedict Spinoza, in Gutman, 1949). Life is the entire state of the living thing, and as an element of human autonomy it is the state of a person which he or she experiences as themselves (Husted and Husted, 1991). In the healthcare setting, if judgement and choice are determined by patient rights and values, then the central theme to that patient's care is their life and well-being. Certain cultural and religious groups view human life as sacrosanct above all else, and feel that everything possible should be done to preserve life for as long as possible, even if the outcome of certain actions may be poor. This may influence patients and carers' views on resuscitation decisions. Tschudin (1992) states that most systems of morality are against killing and are for preserving life. However, she argues that this does not mean that life is life beyond all costs; neither does it mean quantity always comes before quality. Dudgeon (1992) agrees and states that the ultimate goals of medicine are to improve the patient's quality of life, even when dying. Beauchamp and Childress (2001) argue that when the quality of life of a patient is sufficiently low that an intervention produces more harm then benefit for the patient it is justifiable to withhold that treatment. However, they continue by stating that quality of life should be what the patient feels it is, not how the value of that life is seen by others (see also Nagel, 1986). Hayward (1999) argues can it be seen as right to resuscitate someone who, even if the CPR is successful, will die shortly afterwards? He argues at what price does the sanctity of life at all costs have compared to that of death with dignity?

Sometimes prognostic indicators are used by medical staff to see what quality of physical life the patient has. These tend to include the status of the patient's disease as well. There are several types of such indicators. These attempt to state a person's physical state by a score. Numerous ways to measure quality of life have been used, and in a literature review Aspinall *et al.* (2003) found most quality of life measures to be too prescriptive and unreliable. But Costello (2004) feels that measuring quality of health, although difficult, is an important way of developing future services.

The difficult thing about quality if life is it can be a very abstract concept not just based on how a person is physically. Brook (1993) argues that quality of life has three main components:

- human condition in terms of feelings, happiness and satisfaction;
- capabilities in terms of function and performance
- preference satisfaction theory: includes choice, freedom of access and patient autonomy (influenced by culture).

Quality of life includes the actual care given during the palliative stages of a person's disease. Specialist palliative care can provide some of this by ensuring physical symptoms are recognised and responded to; equipment is provided to enable the patient to cope at home for as long as they are able to, or want to; hospice support for day care or admission according to the patient's and their family carers' needs, and the support of understanding specialist professionals involved who have already built up a relationship with that patient.

TRUTH-TELLING

Dean (2001) says that truth-telling shows respect for autonomy. Thus discussing resuscitation with a patient allows venting of the patient's thoughts but also shows respect for the patient by offering the rationale behind the decision. If there is a small chance of success that patient also then has the opportunity to decide, when all the necessary information is given, whether they would want to be resuscitated in their present state and quality of life or not.

In conclusion this chapter has briefly touched on several ethical and legal aspects relating to resuscitation in today's medical world. It can, however, be seen that actual resuscitation decisions need not be complicated by such issues, if dealt with appropriately and sensitively.

9 Resuscitation in the community

This book so far has been more hospital-orientated, although the principles-discussed apply in community settings. Resuscitation status applies in the home as well as hospital, especially if a patient has not had a DNAR order made or discussed with them. For palliative patients who wish to die at home, their resuscitation status must be discussed with them and their carers, so that when the point of death arrives the ambulance is not called.

A resuscitation status made at any point should be ongoing across whichever care setting the patient is in. The patient's health status is a changing situation, from day to day or even hour to hour, and any decision made needs regular evaluation.

The community multi-disciplinary team will usually take the lead from the hospital oncologist or consultant who has been in charge of that care episode as this is where the patient is more likely to have been assessed by a specialist and future care will be advised from there. McCann (1998) stated that the average GP encounters approximately 4.26 cancer-related deaths per year, thus they cannot be experts in this area. However, they still have responsibility as a GP to decide resuscitation status and it should not be seen as a sign of failure if they need to request help from other GPs or hospital specialists in order to do this accurately.

Community staff, such as district nursing teams, Marie Curie nurses, Macmillan nursing teams, as well as GPs, practice nurses, community physiotherapists, community occupational therapists, community dieticians, community carers: all of these can form very close relationships with patients whilst they are at home. The local hospice may also have a close relationship with the patient, either through admission, outpatient or day centre attendance, or through domiciliary visits from doctors or hospice-at-home teams. Visiting a patient in their own home can allow better communication and assessment, with the patient often feeling more relaxed in their own territory and not feeling as vulnerable as they may do in the hospital setting. It also allows a visual assessment of the home and whether the patient and family carers are coping physically at home. Although many deaths occur in hospital, there are increasingly numbers of deaths at home as more government money is identified to use in palliative and community care, and as hospital finances and beds are reduced. The problem again is that in these situations the patient, when admitted to hospital, has a completely different team of doctors, nurses and other professionals looking after them, and giving and deciding their care and treatment. This often results in a lack of continuity and often much confusion about medications and so forth. So although there may be awareness of the difficulty in communication and continuity when patients are discharged home, the same occurs when patients are admitted to hospital.

It is very difficult to see primary and secondary care settings for palliative patients separately since their illness will probably have taken them through several hospital admissions and outpatient appointments (McCann, 1998). All of these care settings will decide treatments and there should be good communication in order to pass on these to each other. However, although many oncology and hospice settings invite community staff to regular multi-disciplinary teams meetings, not all community staff who may have been involved can and arguably, should, attend. Also many other directorates within hospitals will not have such accessible multi-disciplinary teams meetings, although many have community liaison teams who can often access invaluable information from community teams. Many site-specific multi-disciplinary teams now have access to video conferencing, which can allow communication between experts about patients within the cancer network and can share information and expertise about treatments and patient care. Again, these are more hospital-orientated.

It seems so limiting in an National Health Service (NHS) which promises continuity of care, to have such limited communication between care settings. Perhaps, as in some areas, to have staff who rotate between hospital and community (e.g. as do some palliative care nurse specialists) would increase healthcare professionals' awareness of the need to communicate better between teams and would offer the patients better continuity of professionals' involvement. Multi-disciplinary team meetings must cross all care settings to allow a more informative discussion.

The Calman–Hine report (1995) emphasised the importance of good communication between all those caring for cancer patients. Ten years on there has been some improvement, with certain things in place, but this all depends on funding and access to resources. A cancer diagnosis is life-changing, devastating. It is important patients and family carers receive seamless care in order to prevent possible stresses (McCann, 1998). Patients discharged from hospital should take a summary letter to their GP but this has limited information on it, and many are never delivered, and some may not even be accurate due to lack of space for all details of the hospital admission. Consultant letters are sent with more details on them but may take several days, even weeks, to get to the community teams, something GPs have reported include little information on whether the patient understands what has happened to them, and absence of care management plans (McCann, 1998). Resuscitation decisions are not generally included on these letters, perhaps because the majority of decisions tend to be made when the patient's prognosis is only days or hours, and in these situations the patient tends to stay, and die, in hospital. However, many patients may be discharged to die at home, and although a DNAR order was agreed in hospital, the stresses of someone dying at home, or suddenly experiencing a cardiac arrest or sudden collapse, even though generally unwell and frail, may cause the family to call an ambulance. How can this be prevented? It is actually not an easy situation. The lack of communication, sudden acute events on chronic illnesses, family concerns to do the right thing, all can contribute to futile inappropriate resuscitation.

One fairly successful system is called 'Datalink' and consists of a small pot and some small transfers carrying a green cross. The pot is filled with any relevant information concerning anyone in the house, for example recent chemotherapy and side effects, any chronic illnesses such as diabetes or high blood pressure. The pot is stored in the fridge since this is usually the one thing to survive a house fire. Transfers bearing the green cross symbol are attached to the wall just inside the front door where it can be seen by anyone accessing the house. There is also one attached on the fridge door. This should alert any ambulance staff or on-call doctors to relevant medical information or recent treatment. It would be easy to use these for a resuscitation status: thus if all inpatients and out patients were given one, and it was updated on each admission or appointment (not just cancer patients) perhaps this would reduce some of the confusion and inappropriateness of resuscitation. Certain areas within the UK have received sponsorship by their council and other businesses to allow these to be used free of charge. However, again, it is down to the patient's agreement and enthusiasm. In a recent study of patient-held records (McCann, 1998), although many patients found them useful, up to 14% did not like the responsibility of carrying them and 20% did not like the fact they often had to prompt doctors and nurses to fill them in. However, for many patients they are a true record of factual information about their present health status, care plans and treatment management, and most patients may enjoy the feeling of having some sense of control and responsibility in their care.

Some patients choose to use Medi-Alert bracelets or necklaces which alert the attending healthcare professional to an existing medical disorder. This could perhaps include the DNAR decisions, but would be expensive and take time to complete. It would not be funded by the NHS.

Macmillan Cancer Support has recently set up the Gold Standards Framework (GSF) (Macmillan Cancer Relief, 2003) for palliative patients within the community. This was set up by Dr Keri Thomas, a Macmillan GP, who had identified recurring problems with community based-palliative care provision: 'I was visiting lots of practices and asking about the common barriers to providing good care for people with cancer,' says Keri. 'They were struggling with the same issues: communication breakdowns, symptom management, out-of-hours care, and how best to support patients and carers. Studies confirmed that half of all cancer patients die in hospitals, even though most would prefer to die at home, yet some admissions are preventable.'

In response to these findings, Keri brought together a group of medical professionals to discuss the ideal model of care for patients living at home. The GSF, supported by Macmillan and the Cancer Services Collaborative, is the result.

At the heart of the framework are seven concepts, relating to key aspects of palliative care, and tools to enable primary care teams to:

- work as a team and ensure continuity of care
- plan in advance for developments in a patient's illness
- provide patients with the best symptom control
- give support to patients and carers.

These 'gold' standards focus on improving clinical and organisational knowledge and the human dimension of service delivery:

- *Communication*: A Supportive Care Register is used, where all patients appropriate for the GSF are listed.
- *Co-ordination*: A nominated co-ordinator oversees the process of updating information and making sure all care is based on physical, emotional, psychological, spiritual, intellectual areas (PEPSI).
- *Control of symptoms*: Good support to allow accurate assessment and review of any symptoms and medication given.
- *Continuity in out-of-hours care*: Information about patients is transferred to out-of-hours services to reduce crises and support other community staff.
- *Continued learning*: Nurses and doctors are required to make practice and personal development plans, in order to keep themselves up to date with palliative care issues.
- *Carer support*: To support, listen to, and keep the family carers up to date; also to give them practical and psychological support.
- *Care in the dying phase*: To use tools such as the Liverpool Care Pathway, to stop non-essential medications, to use other support mechanisms such as Marie Curie nurses and hospice at home teams.

The framework was originally piloted and evaluated in 100 GP practices and has now been rolled out across the all GP practices within the UK. It has been evaluated to show that it dramatically improves patients' experiences of care, can positively impact on hospital admission and waiting times, can improve staff morale and improve communication between all multi-disciplinary team members. An information booklet is given to the patient and family carers which includes a personal medication record card, information on who is who, and a list of useful contact numbers such as GP, district nurse and Macmillan nurse. At the GP practice, there are regular meetings to discuss the patients on the Supportive Care Register, and to update the whole team on the present situation. Certain templates included in the framework are updated and passed on to on-call teams following these meetings.

This shows there are certain influences in place to try and prevent inappropriate resuscitation in the community setting. However, what happens in the meantime from the paramedics' point of view if they are called to a palliative care patient to resuscitate them, or when presented with a collapsed patient who they feel may have had a DNAR order made but those present do not mention it when asked, or are not aware of it?

In the Recognition of Life Extinct (ROLE) (Joint Royal Colleges of Ambulance Liaison Committee, 2003) paramedics and ambulance teams are given the following guidance in terms of resuscitation.

- *When not to start resuscitation:*
  - decapitation
  - massive head destruction
  - massive injuries – incompatible with life
  - decomposition or putrefaction
  - incineration: full-thickness burns with charring greater than 95% of body surface
  - hypostasis (pooling of blood in congested vessels: indicative of death)
  - rigor mortis.
- *When to discontinue attempted resuscitation*
  - submersion for longer than an hour
  - presence of a DNAR order or a Living Will
  - when all these exist: >15 minutes onset of collapse; non-shockable rhythm on ECG; no bystander CPR prior to ambulance arrival; asystole >30 seconds on ECG monitor.

The European Resuscitation Council (1998) adds

- evidence of cerebral damage
- potential prognosis and underlying disease
- hypothermia: CPR should be attempted for longer
- drug intake before cardiac arrest: sedative, hypnotic or narcotic drugs are said to provide a degree of cerebral protection if taken before the arrest, and prolonged resuscitation attempts are justified.

WHAT TO DO AFTER DEATH IS DIAGNOSED

In bold type the document (JRCALC, 2003) states:

> In patients with cardiopulmonary arrest vigorous resuscitation attempts must be undertaken whenever there is a chance of survival, however remote. However, it is possible to identify patients in whom there is absolutely no chance of survival and where resuscitation would be both futile and distressing to relatives, friends

and healthcare personnel and where time and resources would be wasted in under-taking such measures

However, it is not always easy to identify on attending a crisis situation. The document also states: 'If a family practitioner or third party (relative or close friend) insists on resuscitation then resuscitation should be attempted'. If the GSF is in place in a GP surgery this may reduce the chance of inappropriate resuscitation, but only if the GP on call is aware of the call-out. At present local ambulance stations and police stations are not given the same GSF information. With the increase of on-call doctors covering several different surgeries and areas, there is less ability to access patient records and thus to be aware of each patient's situation. They may easily insist the patient be resuscitated especially if the family insist on this as well and if no resuscitation status has been decided. However, resuscitation can be discontinued once a signed DNAR order relating to the present problem is shown or a Living Will (as long as the family present it). When the patient being resuscitated arrives in A + E it may be possible to access their medical notes quickly (if being treated in their local area) in order to decide about the appropriateness of emergency treatments.

If the patient regains consciousness or is admitted unwell and has not experienced a cardiac arrest McClain and Perkins (2003) state that they should be cared for as appropriate for a patient with a terminal illness, even in the A+E setting. This should include symptom control and patient advocacy, until a more suitable area of care can be found and the patient transferred or until the patient dies.

The resuscitation guidelines (BMA *et al.*, 2001) do state that CPR should not be attempted on transferring palliative care patients to the hospice or home, *Unless the patient or family carer insists.* Yet again, another possible contradiction in these guidelines. However, if a signed DNAR order is shown to the ambulance men transferring that patient they should not attempt resuscitation even if the family carers insist: remember the family carers may not agree with the DNAR order and once out of the hospital they may try to change this. Legally they cannot. It is no wonder resuscitation is attempted as often as it is, a kind of 'cover yourself' issue, with many healthcare professionals frightened in case of litigation.

This again returns to the issue of communication, truth-telling so that the relatives are aware and better patient information. If a DNAR order is made it should be explained to the patient and family in order to reduce any chance of inappropriate resuscitation. Surely if an appropriately made DNAR order is in place there should be no room for litigation from the family. Grief and bereavement can affect carers differently and one coping mechanism often used is blame, thus there may be a desire to pursue litigation. If the success in such cases ceases, the fear of this would be decreased, allowing the multi-disciplinary team to make decisions for the correct reasons and to communicate these to the patients, carers and community staff.

Colquhoun and Jevon (2001) have written a book about resuscitation in primary care. In this they state that the aims of modern resuscitation are the same as medical interventions: to preserve life and maintain health. Many victims of cardiac arrest will not survive, and these patients and their relatives are often exposed to an undignified and perhaps unnecessary procedure with no benefit. They give the success rate of resuscitation when witnessed in hospital between 2% and 20%, emphasising the fact that resuscitation is inappropriate for many of those patients resuscitated. In those whose circulation is initially restored, around 30% of them die later in hospital and resuscitation can be viewed as an extension of the process of dying, imposing considerable suffering for the patient and their relatives. They state that a further proportion of survivors suffer neurological disabilities or other adverse consequences.

On cardiac arrests outside hospital, Colquhoun and Jevon (2001) continue to discuss success rates: this is usually a sudden event occurring in people who are previously well; in such an emergency, immediate action is required and in many cases the likelihood of success, the previous health and quality of life of the patient and the wishes of the patient and their relatives are unknown thus resuscitation is carried out. They state that the main obligation on those who might attempt the resuscitation of such patients should be to decide in advance where a DNAR order is required (where resuscitation is futile) and to use this to prevent inappropriate resuscitation in the community.

The authors state that in their experience problems often arise when staff in nursing homes, residential homes or community hospitals initiate inappropriate resuscitation attempts. The situation is confounded by the ambulance staff who are duty bound to continue resuscitation attempts until orders to the contrary have been issued and this may mean summoning a doctor to attend or by transporting a patient to the local A+E department with resuscitation in progress. A similar situation arises when relatives of a terminally ill patient summon the ambulance when the patient dies, perhaps because of a perception that agonal respirations or gasps indicate that the patient is distressed: a conscious decision not to resuscitate such a patient which has been discussed with family carers can prevent thus situation.

Colquhoun and Jevon (2001) continue that the overall decision for a DNAR order lies in the community with the GP in charge of that patient's care. They will usually be best-placed to consider the most important aspects of the patient's condition and to take into account the views of the patient but need to consider the views of other included multi-disciplinary team members. This DNAR needs to be recorded and signed by the same GP, in order to legalise the decision.

Once a terminally ill patient reaches home for terminal care, the aims should be to continue good palliative care by using the principles of palliative care and providing the necessary carers and equipment needed in order to maintain as safe and helpful an environment as possible. Physical care can be provided by carers, Marie Curie nurses and district nursing teams and includes washing and dressing, pressure area care, bowel care, skin care, mouth care, care of fungating tumours and wounds, dietary advice and symptom control. Community Macmillan nurses and hospice at home teams can provide 24-hour symptom control advice. Often, community support can be overwhelming with many different people involved, as in hospital. It is important in all care settings to appoint a key worker (NICE, 2004) in order to co-ordinate care.

Care should also be directed to the carers, as outlined in the GSF. The patient is part of a social unit and all social roles in this unit will be challenged by the patient's illness, such as breadwinner, parent, spouse, child, friend. Support to the carers includes help and advice over practical issues, such as how to cope with a stoma, dressings, pressure area care, bowel and mouth care, and who to call in certain situations. Other practicalities include to support the carer through any financial issues, physical help, equipment, day care (e.g. at the local hospice), outpatients with specialist palliative care consultants, and when to transfer to a local hospice if required. It can be difficult when hospice admission is most appropriate as most hospices now offer only short-stay beds and timing when someone has only a few weeks or days left can be difficult. However, professionals can only assess according to the situation as they see it and should refer to the hospice if and when they feel it is needed.

Colquhoun and Jevon (2001) conclude that the ethical principles underlying such resuscitation decisions in the community are not much different to the ones used in hospital, but are applied in a special situation characterised by limited time, a lack of accurate diagnostic information, limited therapeutic possibilities and a severely curtailed relationship between the patient and healthcare providers. They state:

> The same principle of providing treatment to preserve life, restore health and the relief of suffering remains, as does the principle of avoiding procedures with potential adverse consequences. The principles of patient autonomy and consent remain even though the patient may be unable to communicate their wishes at the time.

10 The future of resuscitation

Although since the advent of the resuscitation guidelines and mandatory local cardiopulmonary resuscitation (CPR) policies, the approach to resuscitation has started to change. There is now a greater emphasis on openness, honesty and patient choice. However, there is still a lot of room for improvement. The patient's journey crosses many care areas, each with its own multi-disciplinary teams, ideas and experience. Communication is often late, lacking in facts and unclear. This is the same for resuscitation decisions. There are few, if any, hospitals or community practices which, when a patient is transferred to another area of care, will communicate their resuscitation decision. This does tend to happen for patients being transferred to hospice care from hospital, or to home for terminal care, where a signed DNAR form can be seen by the ambulance staff. However, there is often little communication of resuscitation decisions of palliative patients who may not be appropriate for resuscitation but are not imminently terminal and are discharged to the community setting. In hospital, if patients deteriorate a resuscitation status should be considered; however, the GP and community staff are often left without the expertise of the specialist and may be undecided about what to do.

For patients who may suddenly deteriorate and collapse at home, if resuscitation has not been discussed with the relatives, they may call an ambulance and even request resuscitation because they are not aware of why they should not. As seen before, paramedics have a duty to resuscitate except in extreme circumstances.

The future may lie in patient-held records, whereby a resuscitation status could be made, discussed with the patient and written down in these records, which the patient would keep with them. Some patients find such records bulky and are often too intimidated to ask for a doctor to update them on each admission or clinic appointment (McCann, 1998). Another example which has been used quite successfully in the community (as mentioned before) is Datalink, which can then communicate any information such as diabetes, high blood pressure, recent chemotherapy and even a resuscitation decision quickly and easily. It is inexpensive, easy to sort out and not bulky or complicated.

The Gold Standards Framework (GSF), initiated by Macmillan Cancer Relief across the community setting, is designed to include all patients with a

DS1500 form, that is, prognosis can be reasonably expected to be six months or less. Such patients are palliative and the care given to them in the community is based around palliative principles, and treatment aims and decisions are passed to out of hours on-call teams, in order to help reduce confusion and inappropriate treatment decisions. It is important that any information about the patient be effectively communicated by the experts to those in different care settings. This applies to all aspects of patient care, not just resuscitation.

So, patient-held records, GSF and Datalink are very good ways to communicate important information, including resuscitation decisions. However, they can only be helpful if they are used.

Conclusion

This book has given the reader just a taste of what resuscitation and palliative care involves. The subject is huge and readers are recommended to investigate any issues discussed further if they wish to do so. There is so much information available that this book has tried to cover the main issues and information in order to give a taster: to have included all the information would have been an impossible task, and made the book too large to publish.

Resuscitation has evolved to become a very technical area of patient care, but one which is very complex. It is not as successful as portrayed by the media, and patients and family carers need to discuss it knowing the rationale behind it without medical jargon. It is no longer simply a medical decision, but at the same time is not simply a patient or family carer's decision. If deemed to be futile resuscitation should not be offered as an option for the patient, but should be discussed as to why it is not an appropriate treatment.

Resuscitation is different to active treatment and this difference should be explained so that any patient who has a DNAR order made will realise that all other efforts, where appropriate, will be instigated to keep the patient comfortable. If active treatment is not feasible either, the patient should be reassured they will receive good palliative care. A good death, one of peace and dignity, is then the aim. Communication across care settings is now the main issue for the future, but not simply concerning resuscitation orders. Seamless care is not a simple measure but can be achieved if there is support and concern for the patient and their carers.

Further reading

The author certainly does not wish to take all the credit for this book since much of it is the work of others, simply cited here. For those interested in reading further, she has listed some of the articles she found the most useful on the subject of resuscitation in palliative care. Of course, don't just take her word for it: the list is not exhaustive and some readers may find other useful sources in the References.

- Sweet, S.J., Norman, I.J. (1995). The nurse–doctor relationship: a selective literature review. *Journal of Advanced Nursing* **22**, 240–241. (A good overview of available literature on this subject, and investigates why male doctors may find it difficult to work with male nurses.)
- Dallain, L. (2004). Cardiopulmonary resuscitation in the hospice setting. *Cancer Nursing Practice* **3**, 35–39. (A useful article on the subject which discussed the importance of a CPR policy in hospices.)
- Dean, J.A. (2001). The resuscitation status of a patient: a constant dilemma. *British Journal of Nursing* **10**, 537–543. (An easy to read article which looks at the success and futility of CPR against a good death. It discusses CPR in terms of a five-principle approach to ethical dilemmas.)
- Vitelli, C., Cooper, K., Rogatko, A., Brennan, M. (1991). Cardiopulmonary resuscitation and the patient with cancer. *Journal of Clinical Oncology* **9**, 111–115. (An interesting article on the success of CPR in cancer patients in hospital which states that success is least for those with poor performance status, who spend 50% or more of their time in bed at the time of admission.)
- Safar, P. (1996). On the history of modern resuscitation. *Critical Care Medicine* **Feb**, 24 (2 supplement), s3–s11. (A very detailed overview of the practical development of CPR as it is known today. A good article for those wishing to look into this subject further.)
- Ebrahim, S. (2000). DNR decisions: flogging dead horses or a dignified death? *BMJ* **320**, 1155–1156. (A more cynical view of whether ageism can be overcome in resuscitation decisions. Very interesting and thought-provoking.)
- Willard, C. (1996). The nurse's role as patient advocate: obligation or imposition? *Journal of Advanced Nursing* **24**, 60–66. (Willard has written

extensively not only on resuscitation but also on nurse advocacy. It discusses how nurses acting as advocates assume patients actually need this, and how rights and duties can conflict for the nurse when using advocacy if they are not experienced in this subject.)

- Woodrow, P. (1997). Nurse advocacy: is it in the patient's best interests? *British Journal of Nursing* **6**, 225–229. (This covers advocacy in the same vein as Willard's article and warns of the pitfalls and dangers of nurse advocacy. This is certainly a good article for any student or trained nurse to read who may not be very experienced in patient advocacy, or who simply wants a theoretical basis for this subject.)
- George, A.L., Folk, B.P., Crecilius, P.L., Campbell, P.L. (1989). Pre-arrest morbidity and other correlates of survival after in-hospital CPR. *American Journal of Medicine* **87**, 28–34. (Although a little dated now, this article does make interesting reading in terms of whether success of CPR is actually measurable prior to its occurrence in patients.)
- McNeil, C. (1998). A good death (Editorial). *Journal of Palliative Care* **14**, 5–6. (A short article which is easy to read and discusses what does, and does not, contribute to a good death.)
- Low, J.S., Payne, S. (1996). The good and bad death perceptions of health professionals working in palliative care. *European Journal of Cancer Care* **5**, 237–241. (This examines what professionals view as contributing to a good death. Very interesting reading, which shows that the majority of professionals think that a good death occurs when the patient's physical symptoms are controlled.)
- Field, D. (1994). Palliative medicine and the medicalisation of death. *European Journal of Cancer Care* **3**, 58–62. (An interesting look at how dying has become medicalised as an effect of the industrial revolution, and how it may be able to be changed into something less medical in the future.)
- Thomas, A. (1997). Patient autonomy and cancer treatment decisions. *International Journal of Palliative Medicine* **3**, 317–323. (A good article examining patient autonomy; it argues that patient autonomy is not easy or simple and whether it occurs is down to the professionals the patient is involved with.)
- Dimond, B. (2004). Not for resuscitation instructions: the law for adult patients in the UK. *British Journal of Nursing* **13**, 984–986. (Dimond, as always, writes succinctly and clearly, defining what is legal. She also touches on human rights. Easy to read, enjoyable.)
- National Council for Palliative Care. (2003). CPR: *Policies in Action: Proceedings of a Seminar to Inform Best Practice with CPR Policies Within Palliative Care.* London: NCPC. (Excellent reading for anyone wishing to write a policy on CPR in palliative care. All of the Council's publications are easy to read and easy to order on their website: www.ncpc.org.uk.)
- Willard, C. (2000). Cardiopulmonary resuscitation for palliative care patients: a discussion of ethical issues. *Palliative Medicine* **14**, 308–312.

(Willard writes with exceptional clarity concerning CPR in palliative care and leaves the reader with no ambiguity as to the futility of it in these situations.)

- Birtwhistle, J., Nielson, A. (1998). Do not resuscitate: an ethical dilemma for the decision-maker. *British Journal of Nursing* **7**, 543–549. (An easy article for students and newly qualified staff, which outlines the ethical problems they may encounter when being involved with CPR decisions.)
- British Medical Association, Royal College of Nursing and Resuscitation Council (UK). (2001). *Decisions Relating to Cardio-pulmonary Resuscitation. A Joint Statement from the BMA, RCN and RC.* (www.resus.org.uk) (This is certainly the most important item for any reader to look at, since it is the basis of the book's discussions. Although there may seem to be contradictions, in terms of patient autonomy versus doctors decision-making power, nevertheless they are excellent guidelines which should be read by anyone aiming to write either a local CPR policy or patient information, or who wants to investigate the issue further.).
- British Medical Association. (2002). *Withholding and Withdrawing Life-prolonging Treatments: Good Practice in Decision-making.* London: BMA. (An excellent guide to doctors and nurses about the ethical and legal issues involved when dealing with this sensitive subject in practice. Available to download from: www.gmc-uk.org)
- Hayward, M. (1999). Cardiopulmonary resuscitation: are practitioners being realistic? *British Journal of Nursing* **8**, 810–814. (A very realistic overview of the futility of CPR generally. Easy to read.)
- Jevon, P. (1999). Do not resuscitate orders: the issues. *Nursing Standard* **13**, 45–46. (Jevon has written some excellent articles and his writing is straightforward and to the point.)
- Clark, D. (2002). Between hope and acceptance: the medicalisation of dying. *BMJ* **324**, 905–907. (A very interesting view of palliative medicine. He argues that palliative care may actually be medicalising death because it is beginning to use more medical interventions but under the guise of symptom control. A good article to read for anyone involved in palliative care: it may help to balance views on palliative care, that it may indeed be following medical paternalism.)
- National Council for Palliative Care. (2002). *Ethical Decision-making in Palliative Care. Artificial Hydration for People Who are Terminally Ill.* London: NCPC. (Again, an excellent article on the subject of the use of fluids in the terminally ill patient.)
- Kouwenhoven, W.B., Knickerbocker, G.G., Jude, M.D., James, R. (1960). Closed chest cardiac massage. *JAMA* **173**, 1064–1067. (The article that started it all! Makes interesting reading and reinforces why CPR was invented: for sudden, unexpected cardiac or respiratory arrest.)
- Firth, S. (2001). *Wider Horizons: Care of the Dying in a Multicultural Society.* London: NCPC. (A very informative booklet which all healthcare

professionals would do well to read. It helps the reader realise that their own culture and beliefs are not always the same as everyone else's, and that this is, in fact, more the norm nowadays.)

- Ewer, M.S., Kish, S.K., Martin, C.G., Price, K.J., Feeley, T.W. (2001). Characteristics of cardiac arrest in cancer patients as a predictor after CPR. *Cancer* **92**, 1905–1912. (A very good article on the futility of CPR on patients who experience an expected respiratory or cardiac arrest, that is, from a terminal event. This is the article which helps to clarify whether a person should or should not be for resuscitation by stating that those who experience unexpected respiratory or cardiac arrest are more likely to be successfully resuscitated, compared to those who experience an expected respiratory or cardiac arrest.)

- Cooley, C. (2000). Communication skills in palliative care. *Professional Nurse* **15**, 603–605. (Interesting reading about methods of communicating, not just verbal. Useful to all nurses but particularly students and those newly qualified.)

- Herth, K. (1990a). Fostering hope in terminally ill people. *Journal of Advanced Nursing* **15**, 1250–1259. (Herth's work is some of the more respected writings on hope in palliative care. Definitely worth reading.)

- Rousseau, P. (2001). Ethical and legal issues in palliative care. *Palliative Care* **28**, 391–399. (Another good overview article, this time in terms of ethical and legal issues. Very thought-provoking.)

- Bass, M. (2003). Oncology nurses' perceptions of their goals in the resuscitation status of oncology patients. *Professional Nurse* **18**, 710–713. (A small-scale study of how nurses working in an oncology unit view their roles in terms of resuscitation decision-making. Excellent of course!)

References and bibliography

AbuAIRub, R., Fawzi, F. (2004). Job stress, job performances and social support among hospital nurses. *Journal of Nursing Scholarship* **36**, 73–78.

Advanced Life Support Course Sub-committee of Resuscitation Council (UK). (1998). *Advanced Life Support Course provider Manual* (3rd edition).

Allmark, P., Klarzynski, R. (1992). The case against nurse advocacy. *British Journal of Nursing* **2**, 33–35.

American Thoracic Society. (1991). Withholding and withdrawing life-sustaining therapy. *Annals of Internal Medicine* **115**, 478–485.

Anastasio, C.J. (1995). HIV and tuberculosis non-compliance revisited. *Journal of the Association of Nursing in AIDS Care* **6**, 11–23.

Andrews, M., Bell, E.R., Smith, S.A., Tischler, J.F., Veglia, J.M. (1993). Dehydration in terminally ill patients: is it appropriate in palliative care? *Postgraduate Medicine* **93**, 201–208.

Andrews, M.A., Boyle, J.S. (eds). (1999). *Transcultural Concepts in Nursing Care.* Philadelphia, PA: Lippincott & Wilkins.

Andrews, M. (2000). Transcultural perspectives in the nursing care of children and adolescents. In: Andrews, M.A., Boyle, J.S. (1999). *Transcultural Concepts in Nursing Care* (3rd edition). Philadelphia, PA: JP Lippincott.

Animax. (2004). History of resuscitation (www.alber.co.uk).

Argyle, M. (1992). *The Psychology of Interpersonal Behaviour* (4th Edition). Harmondsworth: Penguin.

Aspinall, F., Addington-Hall, J., Highes, R., Higginsons, I.J. (2003). Using satisfaction to measure the quality of palliative care: a review of the literature. *Journal of Advanced Nursing* **42**, 324–329.

Averill, J.R., Catlin, G., Chon, K.K. (1990). *Rules of Hope*. New York, NY: Springer-Varlag.

Bains, J. (1998). From serving the living to raising the dead: the making of cardiac resuscitation. *Society of Scientific Medicine* **47**, 1341–1349.

Ballew, K.A. (1997). *Advanced Life Support Course Sub-committee of the Resuscitation Council (UK)*. London: Resuscitation Council (UK).

Ballinger, D. (1997). Is it ever acceptable to deceive a patient? *Nursing Times* **93**, 44–45.

Barbato, M. (2003). Caring for the dying: the doctor as healer. *Med J Aust* **178**, 508–509.

Bass, M. (2003). Oncology nurses' perceptions of their goals in the resuscitation status of oncology patients. *Professional Nurse* **18**, 710–713.

Baumann, Z. (1992). *Mortality, Immortality and Other Life Strategies*. Oxford: Polity Press.

Baverman, A. (1991). A viewpoint: medical oncology in the 1990s. *Lancet* **337**, 901–902.

Beauchamp, T.L., Childress, J.F. (2001). *Principles of Biomedical Ethics* (5th edition). Oxford: Oxford University Press.

Bedell, S.E., Delbanco, T.L., Cook, F.E., Epstein, F.H. (1984). Survival after cardiopulmonary resuscitation. *New England Journal of Medicine* **310**, 43–44.

Beeber, L., Anderson, C.A., Sills, G.M. *et al.* (1990). Peplau's theory and practice. *Nursing Science Quarterly* **3**, 6–8.

Billings, J.A. (1985). Comfort measures for the terminally ill: is dehydration painful? *Journal of the American Geriatric Society* **33**, 808–810.

Billings, J.A., Block, S.D. (1996). Slow euthanasia. *Journal of Palliative Care* **12**, 1–30.

Birtwhistle, J., Nielson, A. (1998). Do not resuscitate: an ethical dilemma for the decision-maker. *British Journal of Nursing* **7**, 543–549.

Blackhall, L.J. (1987). Must we always use CPR? *New England Journal of Medicine* **317**, 1281–1285.

Bonniver, J.F. (1992). A peer supervision group: put countertransference to work. *Journal of Psychosocial Nursing* **30**, 5–8.

Breier-Mackie, S. (2001). Patient autonomy and medical paternity: can nurses help doctors to listen to patients? *Nursing Ethics* **8**, 510 521.

British Medical Association, Royal College of Nursing and Resuscitation Council (UK) (2001). Decisions relating to cardio-pulmonary resuscitation. A joint statement from the BMA, RCN and RC. (Available at www.resus.org.uk).

British Medical Association. (2002). *Withholding and Withdrawing Life-prolonging Treatments: Good Practice in Decision-making.* London: BMA. Broadway, P.J., Forsyth, D.R., Park, G.R. (1993). The do-not-resuscitate order in the intensive care unit. *British Journal of Intensive Care* **3**, 318–322.

Broekman, B. (1998). Discussing resuscitation with patients: why not? *Resuscitation* **36**, 2062.

Brook, D.W. (Ed.). (1993). Quality of life measures in healthcare. In: *Life and Death.* Cambridge: Cambridge University Press.

Buber, M. (1937). *I and Thou.* Edinburgh: T&T Clark.

Burge, F. (1993). Dehydration symptoms of palliative care patients. *Journal of Pain and Symptom Management* **8**, 454–464.

Calman, K., Hine, D. (1995). *A Policy Framework for Commissioning Cancer Services.* London: Department of Health.

Camarata, S.J., Weil, M.H., Hanashire, P.K., Hubin, H. (1971). Cardiac arrest in the critically ill: a study of predisposing causes in 132 patients. *Circulation* **44**, 688–895.

Castagna, J., Shubin, H. (1974). Factors determining survival in patients with cardiac arrest. *Chest* **65**, 527–529.

Chaplin, J., McIntyre, R. (2004). Hope: an exploration of selected literature. In: Kinghorn, S., Gamlin, R. (eds). (2004). *Palliative Nursing: Bringing Comfort and Hope.* London: Baillère-Tindall.

Cherny, N.I., Portenoy, R.K., Fisher, R.H. (1994). Sedation in the management of refractory symptoms: guidelines for evaluation and treatment. *Journal of Palliative Care* **10**, 31–38.

Childress, J.F. (1982). *Who Should Decide? Paternalism in Healthcare.* Oxford: Oxford University Press.

Chrystal-Frances, E. (2003). Palliative care: a discussion of management and ethical issues. *Nursing Forum* **38**, 25.

Clark, D. (2002). Between hope and acceptance: the medicalisation of dying. *BMJ* **324**, 905–907.

Clark, J. (2003). Patient centred death: we need more innovative research on patients' views of dying. *BMJ* **327**, 174–175.

Clarke, J. (1982). Nursing matters: patient advocacy. *Times Health Supplement*, 19th February.

Cohn, E.A., Leferre, F., Yamold, P.R., Arron, M.J., Martin, G.J. (1993). Predicting survival from in-hospital CPR: meta-analysis and validation of prediction model. *Journal of General Internal Medicine* **8**, 347–353.

Colquhoun, M., Jevon, P. (2001). *Resuscitation in Primary Care.* Oxford: Butterworth-Heinemann.

Cooley, C. (2000). Communication skills in palliative care. *Professional Nurse* **15**, 603–605.

Costello, J. (1995). Helping relatives cope with the grieving process. *Professional Nurse* **11**, 89–92.

Costello, J. (2004). *Nursing the Dying Patient.* Hampshire: Palgrave Macmillan.

Craig, G.M. (1994). On withholding nutrition and hydration in the terminally ill: has palliative medicine gone too far? *Journal of Medical Ethics* **20**, 1339–1143.

Craig, G. (2002). Terminal sedation. *Catholic Medical Quarterly* February.

Cumming, K. (1995). Resuscitation decisions – when should we talk to patients? *Nursing Times* **91**, 40–42.

Dallain, L. (2004). Cardiopulmonary resuscitation in the hospice setting. *Cancer Nursing Practice* **3**, 35–39.

Davies, D.J. (2002). *Death, Ritual and Belief.* London: Continuum.

Dean, J.A. (2001). The resuscitation status of a patient: a constant dilemma. *British Journal of Nursing* **10**, 537–543.

DeBard, M.L. (1981). Cardiopulmonary resuscitation: analysis of six years' experience and review of the literature. *Annals of Emergency Medicine* **10**, 408–410.

Debate of the Age, Health and Care Study Group. (1999). *The Future of Health and Care of Older People.* London: Age Concern.

Deeny, K., McGuigan, M. (1999). The value of the nurse patient relationship in the care of cancer patients. *Nursing Standard* **13**, 45–47.

DeGross, J.M. (1990). Cardiopulmonary resuscitation: how much is it costing us? *South Medical Journal* **83**, 733–734.

Department of Health. (1991). *The Patients' Charter.* London: DoH.

Department of Health. (2000). *Comprehensive Critical Care. A Review of Adult Critical Care Services.* London: DoH.

Department of Health. (2001). *National Service Framework for Older People.* London: DoH.

Diem, S.J. *et al.* (1996). Cardiopulmonary resuscitation on television. *New England Journal of Medicine* **334**, 1758–1582.

Dimond, B. (1995). *Legal Aspects of Nursing* (2nd edition). London: Department of Health.

Dimond, B. (2002). *Legal Aspects of Nursing* (3rd edition). London: Longman.

Dimond, B. (2004). Not for resuscitation instructions: the law for adult patients in the UK. *British Journal of Nursing* **13**, 984–986.

Doyle, D. (1994). The future of palliative care. In: Corless I.B., Germino, B.B., Pittman, M. (eds) *Dying, Death and Bereavement: Theoretical Perspectives and Other Ways of Knowing.* Boston/London: Jones & Bartlett.

Dudgeon, D. (1992). Quality of life: a bridge between the biomedical model and illness models of medicine and nursing. *Journal of Palliative Care* **8**, 14–17.

Dunphy, K., Finlay, I., Rathbone, G., *et al.* (1995). Rehydration in palliative and terminal care: if not, why not? *Palliative Medicine* **9**, 221–228.

Durham, E. (1994). How patients die. *American Journal of Nursing* **97**, 41–46.

Ebell, M.H. (1992). Prearrest predictors of survival following in-hospital cardiopulmonary resuscitation: a meta-analysis. *Journal of the Family Practitioner* **34**, 551–558.

Ebell, M.H., Becker, L.A., Barry, H.C., Hagen, M. (1998). Survival after in-hospital cardio-pulmonary resuscitation. A meta-analysis. *Journal of General Internal Medicine* **13**, 805–816.

Ebrahim, S. (2000). DNR decisions: flogging dead horses or a dignified death? *BMJ* **320**, 1155–1156.

Edwards, S.D. (1996). *Nursing Ethics – A Principle-based Approach.* London: Macmillan Press.

Ellershaw, J.E., Sutcliffe, J.M., Saunders, C.M. (1995). Dehydration and the dying patient. *Journal of Pain and Symptom Management* **10**, 192–197.

Ellershaw, J.E., Wilkinson, S. (2003). *Care of the Dying: A Pathway to Excellence.* Oxford. Oxford University Press.

Elwell, L. (2000). The no-CPR decisions: the ideal and the reality. *Journal of Palliative Care* **16**, 53–56.

Escalante, C.P., Martin, C.G., Elting, L.S. *et al.* (1997). Medical futility and appropriate medical care in patients whose death is thought to be imminent. *Support Care Cancer* **5**, 274–280.

European Resuscitation Council. (1998). Ethical principles on out of hospital cardiopulmonary resuscitation. In: Bossart, L. (Ed.). *European Resuscitation Council Guidelines for Resuscitation.* Amsterdam: Elsevier Science.

Ewer, M.S., Kish, S.K., Martin, C.G., Price, K.J., Feeley, T.W. (2001). Characteristics of cardiac arrest in cancer patients as a predictor after CPR. *Cancer* **92**, 1905–1912.

Faber-Langadoen, K. (1991). Resuscitation of patients with Metastatic cancer: is transient benefit still futile? *Archives of Internal Medicine* **151**, 235–239.

Fainsinger, R.L., MacEarchen, T., Miller, M.J. *et al.* (1994). The use of hypodermoclysis for rehydration in terminally ill cancer patients. *Journal of Pain and Symptom Management* **9**, 298–302.

Fallowfield, L. (1995). Psychosocial interventions in cancer. *BMJ* **311**, 1316–1317.

Farsides, B. (2003). Principles for designing patient information. In: NCPC. *CPR Policies in Action.* London: NCPC.

Faulkner, J.E., DeJong, C.F. (1966). Religiosity in 5D: an empirical analysis. *Social Forces* **45**, 246–254.

Faull, C., Woof, R. (2002*). Palliative Care.* Oxford: Oxford University Press.

Field, D. (1989). *Nursing the Dying.* London: Routledge.

Field, D., James, N. (1993). Approaching death: improving care at the end of life. Cited in: Costello, J. *Nursing the Dying Patient.* London: Palgrave Macmillan, Hampshire.

Field, D. (1994). Palliative medicine and the medicalisation of death. *European Journal of Cancer Care* **3**, 58–62.

Firth, S. (2001). *Wider Horizons: Care of the Dying in a Multicultural Society.* London: NCPC.

Fleming, K. (1997). The meaning of hope to palliative care cancer patients. *International Journal of Palliative Nursing* **3**, 14–18.

Forchuk, C. (1992). The orientation phase of the nurse–client relationship: how long does it take? *Perspectives in Psychiatric Care* **28**, 7–10.

Freud, S. (1925). An autobiographical study. In: Strachey, J. (Ed.) *Standard Edition of the Complete Works of Sigmund Freud, Volume 20.* London: Hogarth Press.

Fusgen, I., Summa, J.D. (1978). How much sense is there is an attempt to resuscitate an aged person? *Gerontology* **24**, 37–45.

Gadow, S. (1989). Advocacy with silent patients. *Nursing Clinics of North America* **24**, 535–541.

Gay, J.E. (1985). Nursing under stress, Part 1. *Occupational Health* **37**(4), 179–183.

George, A.L., Folk, B.P., Crecilius, P.L., Campbell, P.L. (1989). Pre-arrest morbidity and other correlates of survival after in-hospital CPR. *American Journal of Medicine* **87**, 28–34.

Ghusan, H.F., Teasdale, T.A., Shelley, J.R. (1995). Limiting treatment in nursing homes: knowledge and attitudes among medical directors. *Journal of the American Geriatric Society* **41** (Suppl.), SA65.

Gillon, R., Lloyd, A. (eds). (1994). *Principles of Healthcare Ethics.* Chichester: John Wiley.

Glaser, B.G., Strauss, A.L. (1965). *Time for Dying.* Chicago, IL: Aldine Publishing.

Goss, R. (2001). Do not resuscitate orders: without discussion these orders are unethical at any age (Letter). *BMJ* **322**, 105.

Gulati, R.S., Bhan, G.L., Horan, M.A. (1983). Cardiopulmonary resuscitation of old people. *Lancet* **ii**, 267–269.

Gutman, J. (Ed.). (1949). *Spinoza's Ethics.* New York, NY: Hafner Publishing.

Harrold, J. (2002). Palliative care: helping patients and families cope with the ambiguity of dying. *The Forum* **28**, 1–4.

Hartmann, C.R. (1995). The nurse–patient relationship and victims of violence. *Scholarly Inquiry for Nursing Practice* **9**, 175–192.

Hayward, M. (1999). Cardiopulmonary resuscitation: are practitioners being realistic? *British Journal of Nursing* **8**, 810–814.

Helman, C. (1994). *Culture, Health and Illness.* London: Butterworth-Heinemann.

Henderson, V. (1966). *The Nature of Nursing.* New York, NY: Macmillan.

Henley, N. (1973). *Power, Sex, and Non-Verbal Communication.* Rowley, MA: Newbury House.

Hershey, C.O., Fisher, L. (1982). Why outcome of cardiopulmonary resuscitation on general wards is so poor. *Lancet* **i**, 31–34.

Herth, K. (1990a). Fostering hope in terminally ill people. *Journal of Advanced Nursing* **15**, 1250–1259.

Herth, K. (1990b). Relationship of hope, coping styles, concurrent losses, and setting to grief resolution in the elderly widow(er). *Research in Nursing Health* **13**, 109–117.

Herth, K. (1993). Hope in the family caregiver of terminally ill people. *Journal of Advanced Nursing* **18**, 538–548.

Hill, D., Penso, D. (1995). *Opening Doors: Improving Access to Hospice and Specialist Palliative Care Services by Members of the Black and Minority Ethnic Communities*. London: NCPC, paper 7.

Holden, R.J. (1990). Models, muddles and medicine. *International Journal of Nursing Studies* **27**, 223–234.

Holland, K. (2003). Nursing and the context of care. In: Holland *et al*. *Applying the Roper, Logan and Tierney Model in Practice*. London: Elsevier.

Hollingsworth, J.H. (1969). The results of cardiopulmonary resuscitation: a 3-year university hospital experience. *Annals of Internal Medicine* **71**, 459–466.

Honan, S., Helseth, C.C., Bakke, J., Karpuik, K., Krsnak, G., Torkelson, R. (1991). Perception of 'no code' and the role of the nurse. *Journal of Continuing Education in Nursing* **22**, 54–61.

Hughes, D. (1988). When nurse knows best: some aspects of nurse–doctor interaction in a casualty department. *Sociology of Health and Illness* **10**, 1–22.

Husted, G.L., Husted, J.H. (1991). *Ethical Decision-making in Nursing*. London: Mosby.

Iggulden, H. (2003). Communicating. In: Holland *et al*. *Applying the Roper, Logan and Tierney Model of Practice*. London: Elsevier.

Illich, I. (1990). *Limits to Medicine: Medical Nemesis: the Expropriation of Health*. London: Penguin.

Irwin, M. (2001). Terminal Sedation. *Voluntary Euthanasia News* May, 8–9.

Jepson, J. (2003). Do not attempt resuscitation decisions: the nursing role. *British Journal of Nursing* **12**, 1038–1042.

Jevon, P. (1999). Do not resuscitate orders: the issues. *Nursing Standard* **13**, 45–46.

Johnson, A.l., Tanser, P.H., Wood, T.E. (1967). Results of cardiac resuscitation in 552 patients. *American Journal of Cardiology* **20**, 831–835.

Joint Royal Colleges of Ambulance Liaisons Committee. (2003). *Recognition of Life Extinct (ROLE) by Ambulance Staff*. London: JRCAL.

Karetsky, P.E., Karetsky, M., Brandsetter, R.D. (1995). Cardiopulmonary resuscitation in intensive care unit and non-intensive care unit patients. *Archives of Internal Medicine* **155**, 1277–1280.

Kaye, P. (1996). *Breaking Bad News*. Northampton: EPL Publications.

Kinzbrunner, B.M. (1995). Ethical dilemmas in hospice and palliative care. *Support Care Cancer* **3**, 28–36.

Knaus, W.A., Draper, E.A., Wagner, D.P., Zimmerman, J.E. (1985). APACHEII: a severity of disease classification. *Critical Care Medicine* **13**, 818–827.

Kohnke, M. (1982). Myths and realities about advocacy – clinical research-abuse. *J New York State Nurses Assoc* **13**, 22–28.

Kouwenhoven, W.B., Knickerbocker, G.G., Jude, M.D., James, R. (1960). Closed chest cardiac massage. *JAMA* **173**, 1064–1067.

Kreiger, D. (1982). *The Renaissance Nurse*. New York, NY: Harper & Row.

Kubler-Ross, E. (1969). *On Death and Dying*. New York, NY: Macmillan.

Laerdal Medical. (2004). A history of CPR (www.e-mergency.biz/article).

Lantos, J.D., Singer, P.A., Walker, R.M. *et al*. (1989). The illusion of futility in clinical practice. *American Journal of Medicine* **87**, 81–84.

Leininger, M. (Ed.). (1991). *Culture Care Diversity and Universality: A Theory of Nursing*. New York, NY: NLN Press.

Lemire, J.G., Johnson, A.L. (1972). Is cardiac resuscitation worthwhile? A decade of experience. *New England Journal of Medicine* **286**, 970–972.

LeVack, P. (2002). *Making Judgements Based on the Concept of Futility.* London: NCPC.

Levy, D.R. (1985). White doctors and black patients: influence of race on the doctor–patient relationship. *Paediatrics* **75**, 639–643.

Lo, B. (1991). Unanswered questions about DNR orders (Editorial). *JAMA* **265**, 1874–1875.

Low, J.S., Payne, S. (1996). The good and bad death perceptions of health professionals working in palliative care. *European Journal of Cancer Care* **5**, 237–241.

Lugton, J. (2002). *Communicating with Dying People and their Relatives.* Oxford: Radcliffe Medical Press.

Lynn, J., Harrell, F., Cohn, F., Wagner, D., Connors, A.F. (1997). Prognoses of seriously ill hospitalised patients on the days before death: implications for patient care and public policy. *New Horizons* **5**, 556–612.

Mackay, L. (1993). *Conflicts in Care: Medicine and Nursing.* London: Chapman & Hall.

Macmillan Cancer Relief. (2003). *Gold Standards Framework.* London: Macmillan.

Maguire, P. (1985). The psychological impact of cancer. *British Journal of Hospital Medicine* **34**, 100–103.

Mallick, M., McHale, J. (1995). Support for advocacy. *Nursing Times* **91**, 28–30.

Manisty, C., Waxman, J. (2003). Doctors should not discuss resuscitation with terminally ill patients. *BMJ* **327**, 614–616.

May, C. (1995). Patient autonomy and the politics of professional relationships. *Journal of Advanced Nursing* **21**, 83–87.

Mayo, T.W. (1996). Forgoing artificial nutrition and hydration: legal and ethical considerations. *Nutrition in Clinical Practice* **11**, 254–264.

McCann, C. (1998). Communication in cancer care: introducing patient-held records. *International Journal of Palliative Nursing* **4**, 222–229.

McClain, K., Perkins, P. (2001). Terminally ill patients in the emergency department: a practical overview of end if life issues. *Journal of Emergency Nursing* **28**, 515–521.

McGrath, R.B. (1987). In-house cardiopulmonary resuscitation after a quarter of a century. *Annals of American Medicine* **16**, 1365–1368.

McNamara, B., Waddell, C., Colvin, M. (1994). The institutionalisation of the good death. *Social Science Medicine* **39**, 1501–1508.

McNeil, C. (1998). A good death (editorial). *Journal of Palliative Care* **14**, 5–6.

Mendrick, R., Dillon, J. (2000). Fifty elderly NHS death dossier. *Independent on Sunday* 16 April, 1.

Messert, B., Quaglieri, C.E. (1976). Cardiopulmonary resuscitation: perspectives and problems. *Lancet* **11**, 410–412.

Miller, D.L., Gorbein, J.G., Simbartl, L.A., Jahnigan, D.W. (1993). Factors influencing physicians in recommending in-hospital cardiopulmonary resuscitation. *Archives of Internal Medicine* **13**, 1999–2003.

Miller, J. (1991). Developing and maintaining hope in families of the critically ill. *AACN Clinical Issues in Critical Care Nursing* **2**, 229–257, 307–315.

Mitchell, S.L., Kiely, D.K., Lipsitz, L.A. (1997). The risk factors and impact on survival of tube feeding placement in nursing home residents with severe cognitive impairment. *Archives of Internal Medicine* **157**, 327–332.

Morton, R. (1996). Breaking bad news to patients with cancer. *Cancer Nursing* **11**, 669–671.

Murphy, D.J., Burrows, D., Santilli, S., Kemp, A.W., Tenner, S., Kneling, B., Teno, J. (1994). The influence of he probability of survival on patients preferences regarding CPR. *New England Journal of Medicine* **330**, 545–549.

Murphy, D.J., Murray, A.M., Robinsons, B.E., Campion, E.W. (1989). Outcomes of cardiopulmonary resuscitation in the elderly. *Annals of American Medicine* **111**, 199–205.

Myatra, S., Divatia, J., Pathan, H. (2004). In-hospital cardiopulmonary resuscitation of cancer patients: is it worthwhile? *Critical Care* **8** (Suppl.), 2999.

Nagel, T. (1986). Death. In: Singer, P. (Ed.) *Applied Ethics.* Oxford: Oxford University Press.

National Council for Palliative Care. (2002a). *Ethical Decision-making in Palliative Care. Artificial Hydration for People who are Terminally Ill.* London: NCPC.

National Council for Palliative Care. (2002b). *Definitions of Supportive and Palliative Care.* London: NCPC.

National Council for Palliative Care. (2003). *CPR: Policies in Action: Proceedings of a Seminar to Inform Best Practice with CPR Policies within Palliative Care.* London: NCPC.

National Institute for Clinical Excellence. (2004). *Supportive and Palliative Care.* London: NICE.

National Council for Palliative Care and the Association of Palliative Medicine. (1997). CPR for people who are terminally ill. *European Journal of Palliative Care* **4**, 125.

Neuberger, J. (2003). A healthy view of dying. *BMJ* **321**, 207–208.

Neuberger, J. (2004). *Dying Well: a Guide to Enabling a Good Death.* Oxford: Radcliffe Publishing.

New Zealand Resuscitation Council. (2004). History of resuscitation (www.nzrc.nz/newsArchive.php).

Newman, R. (2002). Developing guidelines for resuscitation in palliative care. *European Journal of Palliative Care* **9**, 60–63.

Nursing and Midwifery Council. (2004). *Code of Professional Conduct: Standards for Conduct, Performance and Ethics.* London: NMC.

Nyatanga, B. (1997). Cultural issues in palliative care. *International Journal of Palliative Medicine* **3**, 203–208.

O'Keefe, Redahan, C., Keane, P., Daly, K. (1991). Age and other determinants of survival after in-hospital cardio-pulmonary resuscitation. *Quarterly Journal of Medicine* **81**, 1005–1010.

O'Kelly, G. (1998). Countertransference in the nurse–patient relationship: a review of the literature. *Journal of Advanced Nursing* **28**, 391–397.

Office of National Statistics. (2003). www.statistics.gov.uk

Oliver, D. (1984). Terminal dehydration (letter). *Lancet* **11**, 631.

Orentlicher, D. (1992). The illusion of patient choice in end of life decisions. *JAMA* **267**, 2101–2104.

Oxford English Dictionary, Pocket Edition (2005). Oxford: Oxford University Press.

Page, S., Komaromy, C. (2000). Lonely Death: The Case of Expected and Unexpected Death. Paper presented to the Fifth International Conference on death, Dying and Disposal, Goldsmiths College, London, September.

Palgi, P., Abramovitch, H. (1984). Death: a cross-cultural perspective. *A Rev Anthrop* **13**, 385.

Parsons, T. (1950). *The Social System.* London: Routledge & Kegan Paul.

Payne, S., Seymour, J., Ingleton, C. (eds). (2004). *Palliative Care Nursing: Principles and Evidence for Practice.* New York, NY: Open University Press.

Pearson, A. *et al.* (1997). *Nursing Models for Practice.* Oxford: Butterworth-Heinemann.

Peatfield, R.C., Sillett, R.W., Taylor, D., McNichol, M.W. (1977). Survival after cardiac arrest in hospital. *Lancet* **i**, 1223–1225.

Penson, J. (2000). A hope is not a promise: fostering hope within palliative care. *International Journal of Palliative Nursing* **6**, 407–433.

Peplau, H.E. (1992). Interpersonal relationship: a theoretical framework for application in nursing practice. *Nursing Science Quarterly* **5**, 13–18.

Perakyla, A. (1991). Hope work in the seriously ill patients. *Qualitative Health Research* **1**, 171–177.

Poss, S. (1981). *Towards Death with Dignity.* London: Allen & Unwin.

Printz, L.A. (1992). Terminal dehydration: a compassionate treatment. *Archives of Internal Medicine* **152**, 697–700.

Quill, T.E., Lo, B., Brock, D.W. (1997). Palliative options of last resort: a comparison of stopping eating and drinking, terminal sedation, physician assisted suicide, and voluntary active euthanasia. *JAMA* **278**, 2099–2104.

Quinn, T. (1998). Cardiopulmonary resuscitation: new European guidelines. *British Journal of Nursing* **7**, 1070–1077.

Rachels, J. (1986). *The End of Life.* Oxford: Oxford University Press.

Ramirez, A.J., Richards, G.J.G., Rees, W.M., *et al.* (1994). Effective communication in oncology. *Journal of Cancer Care* **3**, 84–93.

Randall, F. (2003). Ethical considerations. In: *CPR Policies in Action.* London: NCPC.

Raskin, M. (1994). The rope of paternalism in informed consent. *Applied Radiology* **7**, 23–26.

Regnard, C., Kindlen, M. (2002). *Supportive and Palliative Care in Cancer.* Oxford: Radcliffe Medical Press.

Regnard, C., Mannix, K. (1991). Reduced hydration or feeding in advanced disease – a flow diagram. *Palliative Medicine* **5**, 161–164.

Regnard, C., Randall, F. (2005). A framework for making advance decisions on resuscitation. *Clinical Medicine* **5**, 354–360.

Reid, C., Jeffrey, C. (2002). Do no attempt resuscitation decisions in a cancer centre: addressing difficult ethical and communication issues. *British Journal of Cancer* **86**, 1057–1060.

Roberts, D. (2003). Dying. In: Holland *et al.*, *Applying the Roper, Logan and Tierney Model in Practice.* London: Elsevier.

Roper, N., Logan, W.W., Tierney, A.J. (1980). *The Elements of Nursing.* Edinburgh: Churchill Livingstone.

Rosner, F. (1987). Withdrawing fluids and nutrition: an alternative view. *NY State Journal of Medicine* **87**, 591–593.

Rosner, F. (1993). Why nutrition should not be withheld from patients. *Chest* **104**, IR92–96.

Rousseau, P. (2000). The ethical validity and clinical experience of palliative medicine. *Mayo Clinical Proctology* **75**, 1064–1069.

Rousseau, P. (2001). Ethical and legal issues in palliative care. *Palliative Care* **28**, 391–399.

Royal College of Nursing. (1992). *Issues in Nursing and Health: Advocacy and the Nurse.* London: RCN.

Rozenbaum, E.A., Shenkman, L. (1988). Predicting outcome of in-hospital cardiopulmonary resuscitation. *Critical Care Medicine* **16**, 583–586.

Rumbold, G. (1993). *Ethics in Nursing Practice* (2nd edition). London: Baillère-Tindall.

Rumbelow, H. (2000). Patients demand 'living wills' to protect elderly. *The Times*, 14 April.

Safar, P. (1996). On the history of modern resuscitation. *Critical Care Medicine* **24** (2 supplement), s3–s11.

Salvage, J. (Ed.) (1993). *Strengthening Nursing and Midwifery to Support Health for All.* WHO Regional Publications, European Services, No 48. Copenhagen: World Health Organization.

Saunders, J. (2001). Perspectives on CPR: resuscitation or resurrection? *Clinical Medicine JRCPL* **1**, 457–460.

Saunders, J.M., Valente, S.M. (1986). The question that won't go away. *Nursing* **86**, 61–64.

Savage, J. (1987). *Nurses and Gender.* Milton Keynes: Open University Press.

Scanlon, C. (1989). Creating a vision of hope: the challenge of palliative care. *Oncology Nursing Forum* **16**, 491–496.

Schultz, S.C., Cullinane, D.C., Pasquale, M.D. *et al.* (1996). Predicting in-hospital mortality in cardiopulmonary resuscitation. *Resuscitation* **33**, 13–17.

Scott, R.P.F. (1981). Cardiopulmonary resuscitation in a teaching hospital. a survey of arrests occurring outside intensive care units and emergency rooms. *Anaesthesia* **36**, 526–530.

Sepulveda, C., Marlin, A., Yoshida, T., Ullrich, A. (2002). Palliative care: the World Health Organization's perspective. *Journal of Pain and Symptom Management* **24**, 91–96.

Simmonds, R. (2001). *Improving Access to Palliative Care Services for Ethnic Minority Groups.* Progress report for Research Group Meeting, 19 January 2001.

Singleton, J., McLaren, S. (1995). *Ethical Foundations in Health Care.* London: Mosby.

Sommerville, A. (1993). Cessation of treatment, non-resuscitation, aiding suicide and euthanasia. In: Fisher, F., Mcdonald, N.J., Weston, R. (1993). *Medical Ethics Today: Its practice and its philosophy.* London: BMJ Publishing Group.

Smith, R. (2000). A good death (Editorial). *BMJ* **327**.

Stewart, K., Spice, C., Rai, G.S. (2003). Where to now with do-not-attempt resuscitation decisions? *Age and Ageing* **32**, 143–148.

Stewart, W. (1992). *The A–Z of Counselling: Theory and Practice.* London: Chapman & Hall.

Stutor, J. (1993). Can nurses be effective advocates? *Nursing Times* **7**, 33–35.

SUPPORT Principal Investigators. (2001). A controlled trial to improve care for seriously ill hospitalizes patients: the Study to Understand Prognoses and Preferences for Outcomes and Risks of Treatments. (SUPPORT). *JAMA* **274**, 1591–1598.

Sweet, S.J., Norman, I.J. (1995). The nurse–doctor relationship: a selective literature review. *Journal of Advanced Nursing* **22**, 240–241.

Tattersall, M.H. (1993). Hypercalaemia: historical perspectives and present management. *Supportive Cancer Care* **1**, 19–25.

Taylor, M. (1993). The nurse–patient relationship. *Senior Nurse* **13**, 14–18.

Thiroux, J.P. (1980). *Ethics, Theory and Practice* (2nd edition). Encino, CA: Glencoe Publishing.

Thomas, A. (1997). Patient autonomy and cancer treatment decisions. *International Journal of Palliative Medicine* **3**, 317–323.

Thorne, S.E. (1988). Helpful and unhelpful communications in cancer care: the patient perspective. *Oncology Nursing Forum* **15**, 167–173.

Thorns, A. (2000). Resuscitation in palliative care (editorial). *International Journal of Palliative Nursing* **6**, 264.

Thorns, A., Sykes, N. (2000). Opioid use in the last week of life and implications for end-of-life decision-making. *Lancet* **356**, 1866–1867.

Tobias, J., Souhami, R. (1993). Fully informed consent can be needlessly cruel. *BMJ* 1199–1201.

Tomlinson, T., Brody, H. (1998). Ethics and communication in do-not-resuscitate orders. *New England Journal of Medicine* **318**, 43–46.

Tschudin, V. (1992). *Ethics in Nursing* (2nd edition). Oxford: Butterworth-Heinemann.

Tumim Committee. (2001). Medical treatment at the end of life. A position statement. *Clinical Medicine* **1**, 116.

Tunstall-Pedoe, H., Bailey, L., Chamberlain, D.A. *et al.* (1992). Survey of 3765 cardiopulmonary resuscitation patients in British hospitals (the BRESUS study): methods and overall results. *British Journal of Medicine* **304**, 1347–1351.

Twycross, R., Wilcock, A. (2002). *Symptom Management in Advanced Cancer* (3rd edition). Oxford: Radcliffe Medical Press.

Twycross, R.G., Lichter, I. (1993). The terminal phase. In: Doyle, D., Hanks, G., MacDonald, N. (eds). *Oxford Textbook of Palliative Medicine*. Oxford: Oxford University Press.

United Kingdom Central Council. (1998). *Guidelines for Records and Record Keeping*. London: UKCC.

Varon, J., Walsh, G.L., Marik, P.E., Fronum, R.E. (1998). Should a cancer patient be resuscitated following an in-hospital cardiac arrest. *Resuscitation* **36**, 165–168.

Vitelli, C., Cooper, K., Rogatko, A., Brennan, M. (1991). Cardiopulmonary resuscitation and the patient with cancer. *Journal of Clinical Oncology* **9**, 111–115.

Von Gunton, C., Ferris, F., Emanuel, L. (2000). Ensuring competency in end-of-life care. *JAMA* **284**, 3051–3057.

Wagg, A., Kinirons, M., Stewart, K. (1995). Cardiopulmonary resuscitation: doctors and nurses expect too much. *Journal of the Royal College of Physicians* **29**, 20–24.

Waitzkin, H. (1984). Doctor–patient communication: clinical implications of social scientific research. *JAMA* **252**, 2441–2446.

Wakefield, A. (2000). Nurses' responses to death and dying: a need for relentless self-care. *International Journal of Nursing* **6**, 245–251.

Wallace, K., Ewer, M.S., Price, K.J., Feeley, T.W. (2002). Outcome and cost implications of cardiopulmonary resuscitation in the medical intensive care unit of a comprehensive cancer centre. *Supportive Care Cancer* **10**, 425–429.

Wallace, M. (2004). A history of resuscitation (*http://e-mergency.biz*)

Watson, R., Buswell, C. (2001). End of 'a good innings'. *Nursing Older People* **13**, 34.

Way, J., Beck, A., Curtis, R. (2002). Withdrawing life support and resolution of conflict with families. *BMJ* **325**, 1342–1345.

Wheeler, P. (2000). Is advocacy at the heart of professional practice? *Nursing Standard* **14**, 39–41.

Wilkinson, K. (1996). The concept of hope in life-threatening illness. *Professional Nurse* **11**, 659–661.

Wilkins, S., Bailey, K., Aldridge, J., Roberts, A. (1999). A longitudinal evaluation of a communication skills programme. *Palliative Medicine* **13**, 341–348.

Wilkinson, S. (2002). Futility. In: *NCPC. Vital Judgements, Ethical Decision Making at the End of Life.* London: NCPC.

Willard, C. (1996). The nurse's role as patient advocate: obligation or imposition? *Journal of Advanced Nursing* **24**, 60–66.

Willard, C. (2000). Cardiopulmonary resuscitation for palliative care patients: a discussion of ethical issues. *Palliative Medicine* **14**, 308–312.

Willard, C. (2002). *The resuscitation debate for palliative care.* In: *NCPC. Vital Judgements, Ethical Decisions Making at the End of Life.* London: NCPC.

Woodrow, P. (1997). Nurse advocacy: is it in the patient's best interests? *British Journal of Nursing* **6**, 225–229.

Woodward, M. (1998). Caring, patient autonomy and the stigma of paternalism. *Journal of Advanced Nursing* **28**, 1046–1052.

Workman, S. (2003). Doctors need to know when and how to say die (letter). *BMJ* **327**, 221.

World Health Organization. (2002). Definitions of palliative care. (www5.who.iht/cancer).

World Health Organization. (2004). Definition of palliative care (www.who.int/career/palliative/definition/en).

Younger, S.J. (1988). Who defines futility? *JAMA* **260**, 2094–2095.

Yucn, F.K.H. (1986). The nurse–client relationship: a mutual learning experience. *Journal of Advanced Nursing* **11**, 529–533.

INDEX